WIN SOME

DUKE SAMSON M.D.

This memoir is dedicated to
Patricia Celine Bergen M.D., F.A.C.S.

CONTENTS

PREFACE

I n 2013, Mr. Henry Marsh, a well-known British neurosurgeon, published an insightful memoir entitled **Do No Harm**. Composed of thoughtful, heartfelt episodes from his practice life, it's sprinkled with commentary on subjects as disparate as the American health care system, the management of terminally-ill patients, and the specter of his looming retirement. **Do No Harm** is an intensely personal account of a distinguished professional career that offers honest insights into the practice and practitioners of modern neurosurgery in Great Britain. It doesn't pretend to paint an accurate picture of the same or similar issues in the United States. The current collection of brief stories, anecdotes and vignettes attempts to provide that complimentary profile from an almost mirror-image American viewpoint.

Win Some was compiled from several sources, the primary one being my admittedly fallible memory, augmented by a series of personal journals I've kept sporadically over my career. I've included information from three contemporaneously -described events which I subsequently converted into short stories, and from lengthy conversations with neurosurgical colleagues from residency training, the military service, my years in academic practice and from friends around the neurosurgical world. The text itself was composed in fits and starts over a ten-month period beginning in the early autumn of 2017 and ending the following summer.

All chapters except the introductory vignette are arranged in loose chronological order and written in a conversational style as different from that of Mr. Marsh's book as American colloquial speech is from its more formal British equivalent. Rife with slang, shop talk, and occasional profanity, this is the way American neurosurgeons speak to themselves, one another, to their OR teams and on occasion to their patients. Similarly, the chapters' content often varies dramatically from that of *Do No Harm*, reflecting the very different cultural origins of the works. Our two societies are skew in many aspects; for example, the notion of a brain surgeon, armed with a large Old West handgun, making his daily rounds in an English hospital, would be more at home in a Harry Potter novel than a fact-based British memoir.

The vignettes making up *Win Some* are factual; real events involving real people. Many, if not most, of the stories are sad; that's simply the nature of this business. But they're also stories about effort, courage, dedication, and sacrifice; stories about hope, failure, loss, death and worse. They are, above all, a tribute to the incredibly brave patients who willingly entrust the very essence of their lives to the care of imperfect surgeons and a deeply-flawed health care system.

All of the patients in *Win Some* are lightly- and in some cases, heavily de-identified; in addition, I've received direct permission from certain patients or their families -Paul, Marlene, Carole, Lem, Judie, and Chris - to tell their stories, because the stories themselves are so unique as to make anonymity difficult to preserve. On the other hand, well-known medical figures from the worlds of neurosurgery and plastic surgery have been properly identified: these would include Professors Guiot, Tessier, Derome, Yasargil, Heros, Spetzler, Thorton, Odom and Drake, in addition to Dr. Hanes Brindley.

After long thought, I've also anonymized my own practice partners, residents, fellows, and other practitioners using pseudonyms; in a similar fashion, the names and locations of the medical centers, hospitals and emergency facilities in this work have routinely been changed. In those rare situations where my portrayals of individuals have been unflattering, these names have also been anonymized. While these infrequent descriptions are pejorative, their accuracy is corroborated by public information and legal opinion.

Win Some's final pages are a summary of rules of engagement that have been drawn from the professional careers of the best surgeons I've known. The individual rules aren't sacrosanct; however, taken as a group, they describe a behavior pattern that is remarkably close.

CHAPTER ONE

BZ

The sun was still a faint promise behind the oaks lining Soldiers Creek when I opened my front door and stepped out into the tangy smell of a new autumn morning. Early for sure, but my ER shift started at 0700; Sundays were generally pretty quiet and the early morning drive around Washington DC was a piece of cake, but if there were going to be any unpleasant surprises, I liked to have a running start. Plus, BZ was always early.

My beat-up Toyota pick-up slumped at the curb, telling me a stop at the local 7-11 would be critical before we hit the freeway. The front tire's leak was gradually getting worse, but I had no clue when there'd be enough time to get it repaired, much less enough cash to get it replaced. I'd blown out the original on my drive up from Texas; the spare was slick and leaked like a sieve, but Walter Reed Army Medical Center was really busy and the money was tighter than a tick.

My thirteen-month unaccompanied tour at Clark Air Force Base Hospital had ended with a whimper and a week's in-patient stay with me leaking Salmonella from every orifice; being back in the States was a rush, but the cost of two of us living in DC on a major's salary was eating me alive. The bank account was on life support, and I was moonlighting every weekend that I could find a spot.

On the bright side, the District and its Virginia and Maryland suburbs were hospital- heavy, with almost every institution in need of warm bodies to staff night and week-end emergency room shifts. With six years of residency and a busy year in the PI behind me, plus great recommendations from the ER docs back home, I'd had no trouble finding work, although it was no secret that I was much more comfortable in an OR than sorting through the often complex and sometimes nutty patients that wandered into every ER I'd ever seen.

The old pick-up started with only a brief protest and behaved itself on the three-block trip to the convenience store. I over-inflated the tire for good measure, then checked my wallet and put three gallons of regular in the tank, figuring I was at least good for an out-and-back to Olney Maryland. Montgomery General Hospital was located just off I-270 in the Maryland horse country, and as I eased off the freeway and took in the landscape, I thought," Just sweet, really nice." Groomed fields, bright barns and white fences composed a picture book background for the 'estate" homes of this prime suburban real estate. The hospital's grounds echoed the prevalent Federalist theme and pulling into the ER's almost-empty parking area, I was well aware that the only other trucks in sight were attached to upscale horse trailers. Montgomery General was, as far as anyone knew, the only hospital campus in the country to host Sunday meetings of the local fox-hunting club.

"Long way from Mother Parkland and Big D." I grabbed my ruck, checked my watch and pushed through the so-called "Ambulance Entrance" of the ER.

In reality, MGH didn't catch much ambulance traffic, which was one of the two real attractions of the place. The other was the hospital's policy of two physician ER shifts, always pairing a member of the permanent medical staff with a properly-vetted 'moonlighter." Not only did this approach simplify policies and procedures for the part-time help, but it also made certain there was always a doc on the premises who actually knew how to treat a thombosed hemorrhoid or extract a partially-swallowed fish bone.

This precaution was important because the hospital drew almost all of its moonlighters from either the National Naval Medical Center in near-by Bethesda or from Walter Reed in D.C. itself. While this proximity insured an ample, continuous supply of young board-certified physicians who didn't mind working for minimal wages on week-ends and at night, the hospital had learned from experience that high speed, low drag sub-specialty training didn't always include the appropriate management of ingrown toenails and poison ivy. In addition, many of the moonlighters hadn't spent much time in an actual ER in several years. As BZ was fond of reminding me, that's why there was always a real doctor in the house.

I pushed through the empty waiting area, saying good morning to the registration clerk at the triage desk ten minutes before shift change. Once through the double doors into the actual patient care area, I waved at the two nurses charting at the nurses' station and saw my practice partner for the day already inspecting an EKG strip near the bank of monitors. I propped the ruck against one of the physician's desks, then bit the bullet, crossing the floor to where I knew the morning's first lesson awaited.

Dr Balthazar Walsh looked exactly like a "real doctor". A tall, slender, immaculately tailored man in his mid-forties, he wore a whiter-than-white three-quarter length lab coat, complete with stethoscope draped casually around his neck and reading glasses propped on the bridge of an aristocratic nose. The man reeked of medical professionalism. His carefully knotted paisley tie was a muted shade of lavender, his close-cropped hair was tawny brown just flecked with gray and his large eyes were the exact color of faded Levis.

As Walsh arched his brows to look at me, I knew the olive drab scrubs and short, ancient intern's jacket were a serious disappointment. As a rule, I frankly didn't give a rat's ass what people thought of my dress, so I was surprised BZ's disappointment troubled me; an unexpected reminder how much I respected the guy.

We'd worked four previous weekend shifts together; on the basis of that short association, I was pretty sure BZ was the smartest 'real doctor' I'd ever known. Having seen more than my share of ivy tower professors who prided themselves on knowing a whole lot about very little, I could appreciate a guy right in the trenches who relished going hand-to-hand with every disease that walked in his door. BZ obviously loved taking care of people and seemed to know everything about doing it. He was a compassionate human being, a great teacher and an absolute, world class smart-ass who extracted at least a pound of flesh for every lesson he taught. All in all, I thought BZ Walsh was truly the cat's ass. BZ concurred.

"So, look at what stumbled in our door. You resemble something the dog coughed up, soldier. Aren't my tax dollars letting the US Army pay you enough to buy some decent civilian clothes?"

BZ knew exactly how much the Army paid: he'd trained at Reed and been on the permanent staff at Bethesda for five years before "pulling the pin" and joining the private world at MGH. He also knew that my scrubs and lab coat were clean, Army-issue, and all that I had, so switching gears, he held the EKG tracing up." Like to take a look at this little gem, Ace ?"

Reaching for the snaky strip of slick, almost- greasy paper, I tried to make some sense of what seemed to be a completely random scribble wandering drunkenly across the grid marks. Cardiology had definitely never been my 'thing'- I could barely make out both heart sounds-and I probably hadn't really studied an EKG for at least five years. "Let's see- this is really random, like randomly random, right? " Somewhere in my head a distant bell bonged. I caught a faint thread of logic from the misty past and chased it down. "Yeah, but not 'randomly random' but 'irregularly irregular'- no rhyme or reason to it at all, so this has got to be atrial fibrillation, isn't it? Can't be anything else, because if it were ventricular fib, you'd be in there shocking the shit out of the patient, correct?

"Crudely put, Ace- but about what I'd expect out of a white brain surgeon. Actually an orangutan could make the diagnosis of A Fib on this tracing, so that's not what I'm asking you. What's important about this specific EKG? Do we treat it, give this nice little lady digitalis, put in a pacemaker, anti-coagulate her, what? Think! Or is it still a little too early for you?"

I knew to quit while I was ahead. "Shit, BZ- I don't even have a wild-assed guess. I think she's probably going to need to be anti-coagulated at some point to reduce the risk of her forming a clot in her heart and then throwing it to her brain, but does that come first, or something else? I just don't remember."

"What if I told you she just woke up this morning and realized her heart beat was "funny"? That she doesn't have a symptom to her name and just wants to get out of here so she can make the early service at church. What's important here, other than all those squiggles? What does the heart *actually* do? Can you remember that far back?"

"Well, no question its most important job is to pump blood to the brain..."

"Pump, pump, beat, beat, beat! Right- so how fast is it beating? Look at the big squiggles – that's what's important, damn it!"

"I got it-I got it! Ventricular response, right? How fast is the pump beating in response to all that electrical noise, right? So, we count the beats in that space, which is six seconds, and then by ten...so, say a little less than 100, say 95-96 a minute; that's not so bad, especially if she's not short of breath or having any chest pain... right?"

"No shit, Sherlock. We could have *transplanted* her heart in the time it took you to figure that out. So, let's send her to church now and suggest she see her internist Monday or Tuesday. Do you think we should give her some cardiac medication in the meanwhile?

I shrugged." BZ, frankly, I don't have a clue. We both know I was just lucky to have the damn EKG right side up."

BZ laughed and let me off the hook. "She'll do just fine on a little aspirin for the moment. Stick with me, Ace; I'll make a real doctor out of you yet- assuming I don't reach retirement age first."

I told you about the smart-ass part.

It was a medium Sunday, slow early and then the pace picked up around noon. I saw sore throats in kids that probably didn't want to go to Sunday School, two teenagers with bumps, bruises and one decent laceration after a skateboard collision, then a young woman with belly pain who worried me. Belly pain wasn't in my wheelhouse either, but I did remember how to do the work-up. Thirty minutes later I still wasn't sure what was going on.

The girl was tender down in her right lower quadrant, but her lab work was all normal and a flat plate of her abdomen showed nothing but a little gas and a lot of stool. I went back in for a second look, but this time she was so tender I couldn't get her to relax enough to really probe her belly.

BZ stuck his head in the exam door to say that the kid with the laceration was ready for my "surgical magic", so I used the opportunity to introduce him to the young lady and then asked him to "look her over."

Ten minutes later, I was putting the last of several nylon sutures in the wounded teenager when the internist knocked and then came into the so-called 'Laceration Room", a small OR-like room with decent overhead lights and all the surgical instruments the ER possessed, which weren't much. Once in the door, BZ just stood there; I looked up from the needle work to see a disgusted look. Unfortunately, I recognized the expression, and figured the best plan would be to attack. "What? You don't think she's got a surgical belly? She's exquisitely tender right off the mid-line and even though her labs look OK, she's got a good story for early appendicitis. If her white blood cell count was up we'd have to consider that maybe she has the clap, but the way things are, I say she needs a general surgeon to look her over." He shook his head. "What she needed, Ace, was for a doctor to look her over, and obviously I'm the first one that did. They teach you anything at that white bread medical school before you decided to become the next Harvey Cushing?"

"Look, I don't pretend to be some great diagnostician, but I sure as hell recognize an acute abdomen when I see one. I tell you, that woman's cooking something down in that right lower quadrant ..." "You're right, Dumbass- and what she's cooking down there is an egg. Happens to girls like her just about every phase of the moon. The Germans even have a name for it- "Mittleschmerz ", which translates as "middle pain", referring to the approximate middle of the menstrual cycle. Ring any bells?

Of course you took a menstrual history, right? Or were you too shy to ask the lady about her periods? Jesus H. Christ-what else didn't you ask her about, bozo?"

"No, I admit I didn't get a full history, but I know this is the first time she's had this pain and..."

"First time for everything, rookie. The whole picture is so classic that I admit to not even doing a pelvic exam. You do know what a pelvic exam is, right? Or is that too esoteric for you high-powered brain surgery types?"

I'd done a grand total of four pelvic examinations, the last when I'd been an intern eight years earlier. I swallowed but didn't say anything.

"Christ-on-a-crutch! They send me a fool that can't even diagnose Mittleschmertz, much less read a simple EKG, to take care of half Montgomery County for an entire Sunday. I'd be better off with a large animal vet." For the first time he looked down at the wild-eyed teenager. "Don't worry son, this" doctor" can actually sew pretty good- one of his few accomplishments- so your movie star looks aren't in danger. Dr. Samson, see if you can get that dressing on without taping your glove to the wound, and don't bother our lady friend again. She's obviously out of your area of expertise, whatever that might be."

The door closed and the teenager, who'd sat there listening with his jaw gaping, turned to look up at me. "Wow, that brother has a major league mouth on him. He flat ripped you a new one in about thirty seconds, didn't he?"

"Usually doesn't take him that long. He's slower on the week-ends."

"Damn, I didn't know doctors talked like that to one another. He just ate your lunch right in front of me."

"When you're right, you're right. He tolerates fuck-ups very poorly. It's actually a good way to learn, as long as you don't mind the road rash. He's also correct- I do know how to sew, so stay off that skateboard for a week, and you'll be good to go. Your local doc can take these out then or else drop by here some afternoon and whoever's on call will get them for you. Say 'goodbye' to Dr. Walsh on your way out."

The ambulance arrived a little before two o'clock. For Montgomery General, this was a relatively rare event; the hospital was considered a Level Three trauma center, which meant the EMTs were supposed to transport anything that even looked like serious trauma to a higher-level facility, of which there were an abundance. Sometimes trauma just doesn't cooperate.

When the ER doors swung open, I heard a deep bass voice screaming, "Call me an ambulance!" I jerked my head up from the chart I was finishing to see two EMTs struggling with a stretcher overloaded with one of the biggest human beings in captivity. The way the guy's feet dangled over the mattress, he had to be at least 6' 9" and the effort the EMTs were using to move all that meat suggested he weighed in well over three hundred pounds. His massive arms, free of the restraining straps, swung back and forth like the blades of a windmill; the left one caught Beth, the approaching nurse, a glancing blow, and she went down as if she'd been shot. BZ, right behind her, yelled," What the fuck?' and dropped to the floor.

"Call me an ambulance, goddamn it!" The giant struggled to jerk his body erect but the Velcro strap across his chest held tight; only the huge, bloody head lunged up from the stretcher. A fine mist of blood droplets sprayed across the room; I caught some spatter as I jumped up from the desk. Dropping the chart, I grabbed a handful of surgical gauze and ducked a second shower of red stuff on my way to the stretcher, where the injured man was bucking like a rodeo bronc. Despite the desperate efforts of the EMTs, the stretcher teetered on its tiny wheels; I figured we'd all be on the floor in about ten seconds. There was a bloody field dressing dangling from the region of the man's right ear; above it a short scalp wound was spurting with every heartbeat. The guy's entire face and head were covered with fresh blood, but the rest of him was coated with a thick layer of dead leaves. Meanwhile, the arms continued their pendulum -like swings; the lead EMT ducked, yelling "Where?" I pointed at the Laceration Room, running ahead to push open the double doors.

"Call me an ambulance!" The stretcher lurched past, then rocked to a stop under the surgical lights.

Each EMT grabbed for one of the massive arms, while I closed my eyes, pushed through another shower of blood droplets, then none-too-gently dropped my right hand and wrist across the bloody forehead, pinning that big head to the stretcher. The guy looked like a great white shark.

Glancing down at the laceration, then swabbing at it with the gauze, I could see it was ragged, deep and bleeding like gangbusters. To buy a little time, I crumpled up the gauze and stuffed it right into the wound. He liked that not a bit and roared "Goddamn it!", trying to toss his head. I held tight, but one of the EMTs lost his grip and the huge left arm came up like a scythe.

Having had this particular course before, I ducked into the swing, taking the blow on my forearm. When the momentum stopped, I hooked my own arm around the man's bicep, capturing the bloody wrist in my armpit then turning away slightly to secure the wrist lock.

No matter how big it was, this arm wasn't going anywhere for the immediate future. Meanwhile, the second EMT got back in the fight; together they managed to get the Velcro wrist restraint in place. Then I pushed, the EMT pulled and slowly the big arm came down flat beside the bucking body on the stretcher, where we cinched it extra tight against the metal frame.

In tandem we moved toward the other arm, where the lead paramedic was hanging tough; this time with all three of us working, the restraints went on easier. When I stepped back from the stretcher, we were sopping wet with blood.

Naturally, my first back step landed squarely on BZ's bespoke British leather loafer; I heard a muted "Mother...." and then holding on to one anther we did a little dance step around Beth, who was still sprawled on the floor, blinking her eyes and looking around like a newborn. We helped her first to her feet then into a wheelchair Linda had brought into the room. BZ looked Beth over momentarily, glanced down at the giant and grabbed the handles of the chair. He wheeled out into the hall, blurting over his shoulder, "You got this, buddy."

"Right on, BZ."

"I said,' Call me an ambulance'!" The stretcher shook, so I dropped my hands back down to control the flopping head; suddenly the huge mouth turned, jaws snapping shut. I jerked my hands back; the shark analogy was right on. "Jesus," one of the EMTs said, "Did he get you?"

"Not this time, and that's gonna be his last shot. Cut those boots and socks off-let's get a line into this madman, and see if maybe a touch of Vitamin V..." I looked at Linda, who headed for the ER pharmacy on the run.

The giant had veins like pipes; even with the ongoing struggle, the lead EMT was able to get a big bore IV catheter into his foot on the first stick. By the time the IV was running and the plastic catheter had been double taped in place, the nurse was front and center, holding out a small syringe filled with a light gold- tinged fluid. Diazepam, marketed under the trade name Valium, is a short-acting benzodiazepine which targets the central nervous system and had originally been developed for the control of epileptic seizures. Unlike most agents which suppressed brain activity, it has very little effect on respiratory drive and is relatively safe for use in most emergency situations. It has saved many an ER doctor's ass.

I hated to give this fool any kind of sedation before I could do an in-depth assessment, but faced with the lunging head, snapping jaws and arms that might come loose any second, that just wasn't happening. I slipped the syringe's needle into the IV port, depressed the plunger, then chased the 2 mg. of drug into the vein with a slug of saline. The benzodiazepine took less than a minute to make the circuit, shooting through the veins, the heart and the carotid arteries en route to the brain. Just that quickly, all the excitement was over, the big head sagging back onto the stretcher. All the medical types cautiously took a deep breath. We could barely hear the deep mumble: "Call me an ambulance."

I stood up, stretched and looked at the bloody head. "OK, buddy, you're an ambulance... but what the hell happened to you?" Giving the partially-full syringe off to Linda, I raised an index finger to say, "Don't go anywhere with that." She nodded, as the lead EMT stepped away from the stretcher and looked at me.

"Doc, we don't know shit. We got this STAT call from a woman screaming that her husband cut himself with a chain saw and was bleeding to death. We showed up, this guy was lying under a huge dead limb, right next to a chain saw that had cut itself into the lawn. His head and chest were covered with blood, he was breathing but moving nothing. Eyes closed, not responding to anything. We got the limb off him and he had a BP and pulse, so we loaded him for transport. You guys were closest. On the way he started to wake up, and just as we were off-loading him, the shit hit the fan. You know the rest. Oh, guy's name is Joe- Joe Mayfield."

Linda and Beth, who had returned to the action, finished Joe's admitting vital signs, which looked pretty good. BP up a little, pulse about 110 which wasn't bad, all things considered, and he was breathing about 12 times a minute. The lungs sounded pretty clear, at least to me who was no great shakes with a stethoscope, the belly was soft and we could all testify there was nothing wrong with his arms and legs. I wasn't willing quite yet to turn the guy over to inspect his back, but -other than the head lac - his neck, face and head seemed OK. The scalp wound, about mid-way between his right ear and the peak of his head, had soaked my gauze pack and was still pumping away.

"Head wounds just bleed like stink, but this nick won't kill old Joe here. I'm going to pack it again for a minute while we try to figure out what's going on inside his head. If it bleeds too much I'll put some staples in it. Hell, I'll get you to do that, Beth- payback is a mother."

BZ, who'd arrived silently, looked down over my shoulder. "That Valium really chilled him out. Maybe we better fix that lac before he comes back to join us. These two guys have got to get back on the road, so pretty quick we're going to be down to just you and me and the nurses if he wakes up."

"I hate it when you're right, BZ. In this big dude, that dose of valium will wear off pretty quick. So let's just stick two or three staples in there now and then I can do a plastic closure later after the smoke clears. Linda, you want to get one of those skin staplers for me?"

I washed the wound out with saline and could see a small artery pumping on both sides of the ragged laceration. Using a hand on each side of the cut, I pushed, bringing the lips of the wound together. "Beth, just press the stapler hard against the skin edges and squeeze the handles together. Probably take about four, maybe five staples to close it up."

She held the plastic device in both hands and squeezed. "Kerchunk-Kerchunk-Kerchunck –Kerchunk." The wound closed, the bleeding ebbed to a slight trickle almost immediately and the injured man only grunted. I turned the head loose and stood to stretch my back. Something didn't seem quite right.

"I actually thought we'd get more out of him than that. Those little staple bastards hurt like hell for a second."

As if reading my mind, Joe began to move again, slowly wagging his head from side to side and straining against the restraints. The EMTs were ready to body slam him again, but I said, "Hold off for a minute." Eyes still closed, Joe muttered, "Call me an ambulance." I watched him squirm on the table for a moment, then shook my head. "Oh, shit."

BZ started out the door, but stopped, puzzled." What's up with you, Ace? We need to get this gentleman cleaned up, worked up and ready to send someplace more appropriate. They can sew up his head at Elsewhere General."

I ignored him. "Take the restraints off, guys- all of them, right now."

The nurses and EMTs looked uncertainly at me and then at BZ who had turned and walked back to the side of the stretcher. I said, 'Just do it.'

The Velcro straps came off a lot easier than they'd gone on, and as they released, Joe's arms and legs began to move. The EMTs stepped out of arm's reach, but I leaned over the right side of the stretcher. BZ knew there was something he was missing, but had no clue." We got a problem, Ace?"

"Look- He's not moving that left side much, neither his arm nor leg."

BZ moved up close and after several seconds agreed." No question, he's weak on the left. Was he that way before you hit him with the Valium?"

"Hell no, he almost took my head off with that arm before we got him tied down. It's not the drug- he's got something going on in his head- and it's getting worse in a hurry."

BZ shook his own head. "You think it's a stroke, or what?"

"I think he's got a skull fracture and a clot in there that's getting bigger as we speak. Head trauma, loss of consciousness, then confusion and now a hemi-paresis. Pretty textbook for an epidural hematoma." I nodded, looking up at him.

BZ was smart and proud of it- he hated not knowing things, and hated admitting it worse. Especially to someone he considered a student. After a few seconds and a deep breath, he said," Ehh, well…being an internist and all, I may have forgotten all that I ever undoubtedly knew about these hematomas. So, what's this epidural bullshit?"

"So, you get a hard lick on the head, and the force bends this thin part of the skull in until it cracks. The crack tears an artery in the membrane that covers the brain; you probably remember we call that the dura. The artery bleeds like shit-just like that artery in the scalp- and a blood clot starts to collect. Because it can't expand out- the skull's not going to move- it begins to expand inward and crowd the brain. The brain's just the consistency of jello, so pretty quick it gets compressed, and just stops working. If the clot gets big enough to start putting pressure on the brain stem, it doesn't take long before the patient loses consciousness, then stops breathing. Party's over."

Disbelief. "So you're telling me he's not moving his left arm and leg because there's a clot's pressing on the other side of the brain?"

"Well, it's probably a little more complicated than that. If the pressure on the brain directly underneath the fracture causes that area of the brain to stop working, the arm and leg on the opposite side of the body go out. Alternatively, the brain can be shifting away from the mass of the clot fast enough that the brain stem, which is down deep, smacks up against the bone down at the skull base. Then, the first thing that stops working is the nerve bundle in the stem that controls the arm and leg on the *other* side of the body, meaning the same side as the clot's on. Little bit of a diagnostic problem."

BZ was getting wound up. "So how the fuck do you brain surgery geniuses figure out which side the clot is on- or if there even is a clot?"

"Usually, we've at least got a skull x-ray, which most times will show us a fracture, then maybe a CT scan to actually show us the clot. Right now, we don't have either, and it looks like there's not enough time to get anything."

"Jesus H. Christ! You mean you're just guessing?"

"No, this all pretty classic. If I'm right, one of his pupils will be really dilated because of the pressure on that nerve down at the brain stem. The clot'll be on the side of the big pupil...most of the time."

"Listen to me, Captain America- we need to get this dude right back in that ambulance and over to some place that..."

"I wish, but he'll be long dead before he gets anywhere, much less before they find a neurosurgeon to see him."

"Samson, I really don't like where this is going. What are you saying?" "If we don't fix him here, he isn't going to get fixed, BZ."

"Just for fuckin' starters, Ace, this is not a neurosurgery hospital-there's never been a neurosurgery case even done here. There are no neurosurgery instruments in this non-neurosurgery hospital and if there were, we couldn't get them because the goddamn non-neurosurgery operating room is locked on the fucking week-end. Furthermore, you definitely do not have operating privileges here-hell, I don't even have operating privileges here- you're just a damn moonlighting ..."

"Right, damn moonlighting neurosurgeon... and I'm going to crack this guy's head right here in your ER. Right now, before he's dead."

"What, pray tell, if you're wrong? You're not a stranger to being wrong, as I recall. What if there is no clot?"

"Then he's fucked –and we're fucked."

"No, *I'm* fucked, Ace. You're in the goddamn Army - I actually work here, or at least I will until tomorrow."

"BZ, he needs to have that clot out, or he's toast. You figure out the rest of it- you're getting the big bucks."

Standing on either side of Joe, we looked at each other for what seemed like minutes. Then BZ broke the stare, and shook his head. "Shit. Linda, get Beth in here. And shut that damned door."

The EMTs started for the exit, but BZ held up one palm. "Stand down, you two; we're going to need all the manpower we can get, and probably more than that. Put some gloves on and do what Dr. Samson here tells you."

I stepped over to Joe's head and used my index fingers to pry apart the lids of his left eye.

"First, let's see what his pupils tell us. Beth, angle that overhead down here so we get a look – this pupil looks normal, about 4mm in size and it's reacting to the light." I rotated Joe's head so that the right side of his face was now under the overhead and separated the eyelids again. After a quick peek, I looked up at BZ.

"You want to see, before we go ahead?"

BZ nodded and leaned around my body, adjusting his bifocals to look down at Joe's face. He glanced away and then bent over more deeply, peering through my fingers.

"That pupil is very large, and it's not responding at all to the light. Let me see the other one. OK, I got it- Beth, move that light for a moment."

He turned back. "OK, even a blind hog will occasionally find an acorn. So, even if you're right, what are you going to use to get inside that skull? We'd better have it right here in this very ER, or you're S.O.L. Sterile Supply is locked up tighter than a duck's butt."

That question had been hammering my brain like a rabid woodpecker since I'd first realized where Joe and I were headed. I'd run through every theoretical combination of available instruments I could imagine, and finally decided we had one possible shot.

"BZ, we've got a chest tray down here, don't we? You know, one of those sets the thoracic guys use for putting in chest tubes?"

"Damn right, but it ain't got no drill, just that big ugly... "He paused and squinted a question at me. "Trocar?"

"Yep."

The chest trocar resembles nothing so much as a large stainless-steel screwdriver with its tip filed to a single sharp point. Used to punch through the chest wall between ribs, it makes a hole that looks like a point-blank encounter with a spear gun.

"If there's a fracture line in the temporal bone, I think we can get the tip of that trocar in there and then..."

"Ain't no "we" about this, Ace. In the US Air Force, they'd refer to this as a "solo mission.""

While the two nurses opened the chest tray on a small stand by Joe's head, BZ worked to stuff a plastic nasal cannula down through his nose and into his upper airway. Joe didn't protest much, even when BZ used the suction apparatus to clear out blood and mucous from his throat.

"This cat's pretty far gone, Dr Samson. You better do some of that shit-hot brain surgery stuff pretty quick or this is just going to be a partial autopsy."

I turned Joe's head to the left and elevated it on folded sheets, then grabbed the lead EMT's hands and placed one on the forehead and the other just behind Joe's right ear." You need to really hold him tight; he's going to try to come off the table if he's got anything left".

I poured a pint of iodine solution over the head and the EMT's hands, then changed gloves and took the plastic- handled scalpel from the tray, turning it over so the blunt side of the blade was down. Using only the blade's point I scratched a long thin line, running straight north from in front of the right ear up to the stapled wound. Joe didn't move.

"BZ, get in here. Put one hand on each side of that line, spread your fingers and bear down hard. When I open that incision, it's going to bleed bad for a minute, and your pressure is all we've got for control until I can get a retractor in there."

Looking up at the nurses, the EMT and then at my partner, I muttered," Lock and load." My infantry buddies told me they said that when the shit was about to hit the fan. BZ said, "We're well and truly fucked."

The blade spilt Joe's scalp like it was wet toilet paper. Blood jetted into the long wound, but when BZ unconsciously increased his pressure, the bleeding all but stopped; simultaneously, his fingers caused the lips of the wound to gap open even wider. I stuck my gloved index finger into the incision, undermining the skin to expose the dark red muscle layer beneath. The muscle, bruised and swollen, was so thick I couldn't feel the details of the skull beneath. Targeting the bloody muscle just in front of the ear, I jammed the scalpel's blade straight down until it bit bone. With the tip against the skull, I steadied the head with my left hand and ripped the blade through the entire length of the exposed muscle.

"Whoaa- that's some no-shit bleeding you've got now, Ace."

"Shut up and press harder- I got to get the muscle up before we can get any retraction in there."

I reversed the scalpel and using the blunt end of the plastic handle, scraped the dense muscle away from the underlying skull. Although BZ grabbed the loose suction and stuck it into the wound, there was too much bleeding to see anything, but I felt the handle" tick" across an irregularity in the bone as I scraped it back and forth across the skull. My left index finger probed the wound, and I looked up into BZ's eyes. "At least he's got the fracture."

When the muscle was mostly freed from its attachments, I forced a small skin retractor, taken from the chest set, as deep into the muscle as the small rake-like blades would go. Squeezing the ratchet handle with both hands, I forced the blades to separate very slowly . The skin and muscle opened, exposing ivory skull in the depths of the wound. When BZ's sucker cleared the blood, I was looking at a ragged, irregular fracture line.

Beth said, "Duke, he's not breathing much."

BZ: "Yeah, and this EKG tracing is going to shit as well."

I grabbed the spike-like trocar, steadied it against the fracture line, then tapped the handle with my open palm. Nothing. Swamped by a surge of fear, anger and frustration, I slammed the heel of my hand down. Two inches of steel shaft disappeared into the skull.

BZ winced." Oh, my ever-loving Jesus!"

I torqued the trocar and levered on the handle; an almost circular disc of thin bone the size of a silver dollar popped up out of the wound to land on the floor. I was looking down at a thick tongue of purple clot. "BZ- suck in there, right there, now, now!"

Walsh pushed the plastic suction tube into the clot and we heard what sounded like the sudden flush of an industrial toilet. Startled, BZ dropped the tube but I caught it, jamming the tip back under the bony edge. The clot kept coming out in large, noisy chunks and finally I could see the surface of the dura, pulsating faintly like a weak steel heart.

Within seconds, Joe moved. Beth and the free EMT re-captured his arms and applied the restraints while BZ and the other EMT tried to hold the giant head. In a minute it was like four children wrestling an alligator. I was able to keep one hand on the retractor and the second holding the suction against the dura, but we would have lost control if BZ hadn't rallied in a hurry.

"Linda- where are you, girl? Give this gentleman some more IV Valium before he hurts somebody." A quick squirt, thirty more seconds of all-out scuffling, then Joe went back to sleep and everybody else took a deep breath.

I looked at BZ." We better figure out what comes next real quick. I need to keep this suction up against his dura until you find somebody to get him to the OR, get the bleeding stopped and clean up this mess. Any ideas?"

BZ slowly released Joe's head and stood erect. "First thing we do is get a bunch more Valium in here.

Linda - you watch him like a hawk. 2ccs push, girl, anytime he starts wiggling around. Second, I'm fixing to start another IV. We'll type and cross match him for some blood, then give him a large dose of every antibiotic I can remember. Then, by God, I'm going to call the chief of staff of this pissant hospital, and make him find me a real, certified, no-shit private neurosurgeon, or else my very next call will be to The Washington Post." He squinted at me. " Meanwhile, you white boy, are going to get that bleeding slowed down to a respectable level ; simultaneously, I recommend you start thinking hard about your confession to the State Medical Board."

17

The internist disgustedly stripped off his gloves, tossed them at a can in the corner, pushed his bifocals back on his nose and straightened his lavender tie. Before he could make it out the door, I said, "Hey, BZ."

Dr Balthazar Walsh stopped in mid-stride, turned his elegant head and looked quizzically down his long nose at me.

I grinned. "Fuck a bunch of Mittleschmerz, you dig?"

BZ faked a scowl, took a long deep breath and then smiled. "Well, you can just call me an ambulance, Ace."

The party wasn't quite over, as BZ had a difficult time convincing the hospital CEO that in fact one of the moonlighters had actually opened a patient's head in the ER and now we needed someone to clean up the mess. Turns out there actually were several neurosurgeons on the hospital's medical staff, although none had ever done anything like an operative case there. Ironically, the guy they finally contacted was a genuine knucklehead; I'd met him at a local medical meeting and it was love at first sight. He'd graduated from a second rank program in the area after marrying the daughter of the owner of about forty local appliance stores; just too busy to do any service time, he'd become a conscientious objector. He loved to run his mouth, mostly about money, but the word was he couldn't find his neurosurgical ass with both hands and an anatomy chart. Naturally this clown (Dr. Jaune)was super elated to be called on a Sunday afternoon and told to get his sorry butt to the hospital, but BZ finally had a word with him that turned the tide.

While all this was going on, I was holding a sucker up against Joe Mayfield's dura mater and hoping the pharmacy didn't run out of Valium. After almost two hours, an anesthesiologist showed up and put Joe to asleep for his trip to the OR. I explained what had gone on, and he laughed. "Nice work; I don't know which of you two son-of-a-bitches is the luckiest."

BZ said to him," Just go on and pass your gas, dear doctor, but don't be bothering my man here." " My man," eh? That was a real change, but we still had some work to do.

I went upstairs with Joe, using a portable Gomco suction machine to keep clot out of the wound, and BZ trailed along, ostensibly monitoring the second bottle of blood we'd started, but actually running interference for me with the OR crew, who were having a hard time believing they were going to do some brain surgery on Sunday evening. Dr. Jaune was washing his hands and, believe it or not, avoided even speaking to either of us. BZ said to me, "That's the kind of turd that gives white people a bad name."

Then he stuck his head in the door and called to the surgeon," If you've got any questions, Doctor, I'll be downstairs all night." What a mouth.

I learned two things about our C.O. brain surgeon later, naturally from BZ. The first was that he billed Joe's insurance for $6000 (a significant chunk of change in 1976) claiming he'd performed "an emergency craniotomy with evacuation of epidural hematoma", when what he'd actually done was wash out the wound and sew it up. His other smooth move was to file a complaint with the hospital's medical staff, requesting cancellation of my temporary staff status alleging I had "performed an unnecessary operative procedure without appropriate privileges," proving again there are some people you just can't underestimate. BZ jumped on that one like an avenging angel and the complaint was withdrawn the day after it was filed.

Joe Mayfield must have been indestructible, because he recovered fully without even a wound infection.

Again, according to BZ, he was able to return to work about a month after we'd met him. That was around the same time I got paged to the Hospital Commander's office at Walter Reed to answer questions about my "off-duty" employment. Scheduled to get out of the Army in another couple of months, I figured this couldn't be anything but bad news. To my great surprise, what I found was a nice flower arrangement and a sweet note from Joe's wife who had tracked me down, again through Dr. Balthazar Walsh, just to say thanks.

You can't beat taking care of people. Which reminded me of how I got into this business in the first place.

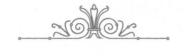

CHAPTER TWO

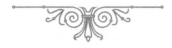

First Things

As an eighteen-year-old kid, I went off to college with an old yellow Ford pick-up and a football scholarship, innocent of any idea what came next once the clock ran out on being a linebacker. Two years later, when I suffered a second knee injury that resulted in surgical removal of all of the cartilage in my left knee joint, I wasn't any wiser. However, lolling around in Stanford's University Hospital during the post-op period, it dawned on me that medicine might be promising as a lifetime gig. My surgeon, a sweet guy, went to all the sports events free, had a indoors job with lots of help, did some operations that sounded pretty cool, and was obviously making a decent living. Plus, there were all these gorgeous young women everywhere I looked. By the end of Spring Quarter, when I came home to Texas for the summer, the knee was OK for straight-ahead walking, but running, rugby and football were out of the question. So, I decided to give medicine a closer look.

During high school I'd undergone a couple of minor surgical procedures at the hands of a well-known orthopedist at a multi-specialist clinic in Temple Texas, so early that summer I gave Dr. Hanes Brindley a call to ask if I could come down to watch some surgery. He said, "Well, let's start with seeing some patients."

So, on the first day I attended an afternoon clinic, where I watched Dr. Brindley and his fellow, a former Rice running back named Bill, as they put on casts and sawed them off, examined hips, shoulders and knees and finally talked with their two patients for the next day's operations. One older gentleman was scheduled for an above-knee amputation; the second pre-op patient was being teed up for a complex hip and femur reconstruction, which sounded to me like an Erector Set project. That evening I had dinner with Dr. Brindley and his family, then bright and early the next morning met him in the hospital's parking lot.

The veteran surgeon (probably late forties) took me up the OR suite to be outfitted with a pair of surgical scrubs, some booties, a cap, a mask, and a locker key. Then, after "gearing up" as he called it, I followed him into his OR where a nurse anesthetist was putting the patient scheduled for the amputation under anesthesia. Dr. Brindley introduced me to the OR team as "ex-football player, potential surgeon", then showed me where to stand once the patient was prepped and draped.

Before he went out to scrub, he had a little heads-up warning for me. "Young man, it's not every day you watch someone get his leg cut off, and there are also going to be some new sounds and smells. So, if at any time you feel uncomfortable or light-headed, don't be embarrassed. Take a few deep breaths and look away for a minute or so. If that doesn't do it, just back out of the doors we came in and go back down to the lounge. This amputation won't take very long; once we're done, I'll come down to see if you want to give the next case a try."

I thanked him for being so gracious but said I was pretty certain I'd be fine. After all, I was an experienced hunter, had been to several cattle round-ups and had done a little first aid training, so how bad could it be? Well, when he and Bill turned the skin and muscle flaps on that poor diabetic patient, "queasy" doesn't quite do justice to my reaction. Then Dr. Brindley started to dissect out the vascular pedicles and Bill, turning so I could have a better view, invited me to come a little closer to the OR table. I already knew the sights and smells up close were going to be more than I could handle, but I was too embarrassed not to step up.

Bill looked at me, then said, "Are you all right?" At that exact moment, the drawstring on my scrub pants came loose. Quick hands for a linebacker-I caught them around my ankles- but for more than a moment or two, there I was in my tighty-whiteys. Bill laughed his ass off (typical ex-running back) but Dr. Brindley just said," That's happened to all of us."

Looking at me, he suggested I retire, recover and re-tie in the Doctor's Lounge. I barely made it out the door before Bill started with the bone saw.

About twenty minutes later Dr. Brindley showed up with a handful of x-rays, a note pad and pencil. Bill had taken the new amputee to the Recovery Room; I wasn't one bit sorry he wouldn't be around for my ignominious departure. Before I could open my mouth, Dr. Brindley was sitting next to me, saying, "This next patient is a really interesting problem; let me show you what her x-rays mean and how I think we can fix her." He was right; looking at the images and then seeing him sketch out how he planned to change things was more than interesting. It was even fascinating.

When we went back in and old Bill slashed the lady open from hip to knee, I didn't even flinch, much less turn green. I was captivated by the layers of anatomy, the way the two men worked in concert to dissect the tissues, stop the bleeding and manipulate the fractures and finally by the drills, bolts, screws and plates they used to hold the whole construct in one tight piece. The triple knot I'd put in my drawstring held, but even if it hadn't, I'd have stayed there in my Jockeys to watch them put this lady's leg together. The following morning I went back to West Texas pretty sure of my next move.

Decisions, especially big, life-shaping ones, are doubly difficult, because they actually come in two parts. First is the decision, then comes the follow-through. Life would be 50% simpler if we all could adopt the old Texas Ranger motto: "Be sure you're right, then go ahead". But absent divine intervention, how in the hell do you know you're right for starters? I believe that's one place where sports are tremendously beneficial to kids growing up, because sports are all about decisions and follow-ups, plus most of that decision-making has to be done without the foreknowledge of what will work and what won't. So, the young jock uses the available information, makes a commitment, then busts his/her butt to make the decision work. But sports also teach you that none of those decisions are guaranteed to be productive; the hooker is, you'll only learn for certain if you've gone all in.

I was fortunate that my college life followed that same, simple trajectory: I decided to play ball until I couldn't, and then -after screwing around for several months-I decided to go to medical school. The "going ahead" part involved working my fanny off for three years to get admitted, which was easier said than done, but there wasn't a lot of dithering around. "Going ahead" has always been less difficult for me than being sure I was right; some psychiatrists will tell you that should be every surgeon's epitaph.

Medical school was almost an exact copy of college; head down, work hard, figure out what it all means as I neared the end. For a lucky minority of my classmates the curriculum was like ice cream, and they loved every flavor. Those fortunate few uniformly did well, but even for them there was some angst in finally picking and choosing their subspecialty career. On the other end of the spectrum, there were a few folks who stumbled on a "passion" along the way, but each of them still had to master the rest of the curriculum to just get a shot at what he or she really wanted to do. Either way there weren't many crucial decisions called for until we all got pretty close to the end.

Post-graduate training was more of the same; we'd each picked our poison and there was more information than one human being could ever absorb in the limited time allotted, so most of us just kept the pedal to the metal, with the realization that, in that era, more than a third of residents washed out. That really wasn't an acceptable option, so we just kept working; in three or four years we looked up to find we'd made the cut and were deep in our final year- about to become "real" doctors. And really, since enrolling in college, we'd only made three or four momentous decisions, all of which were much less difficult than the effort required to realize them.

Beginning with my experience with Dr. Brindley then throughout medical school, I harbored the sneaking suspicion I was destined to end up a surgeon. There was a brief flirtation with Psychiatry, but to me, it seemed there were too many strange folks on both sides of the desk. Cardiology was pretty cool, but unfortunately, I couldn't hear most of the heart sounds, and while I really liked Emergency Medicine, primarily because of the drama and excitement of THE PIT, there was always something about the mystique of the OR, the cunning way those masked men (and then they were all men) used anatomy and dissection and mechanics to try to make patients better. I resonated with the aggressive way they physically attacked injuries, diseases and even impending death; finally, it seemed important to me that they knew, usually at the end of the day, if they'd won or lost the fight. When I just stopped worrying about all the options, the decision pretty much made itself, and off I went to Duke University Medical Center to do my surgical internship.

This was the era of the very first heart transplants, so cardiac surgery was on almost every surgery intern's mind. I think there were sixteen of us in my internship class and ten thought they were the next Denton Cooley. Dr. Cooley was a hero around Duke, because he and most of the Duke surgeons were proud off-springs of the Johns Hopkins tree where Alford Blaylock had pioneered many of the modern cardiac surgery procedures, especially as they applied to children. Duke's current chief of surgery was an arrogant Hopkins alumnus himself, a cardiac surgeon and a strong believer that there was no such thing as overwork for surgical trainees. Consequently, Duke interns were in the hospital 36 out of every 48 hours, for twelve long months. That's known in the trade as every-other-night call, and on-call 'terns spend a lot of that time baby-sitting heart surgery patients.

At Duke or any big university program, cardiac surgery is without a doubt the most visually-impressive of all the surgery specialties. By its nature it requires large teams of three to five surgeons, and a similar cadre of nurses, in addition to a heart-lung machine minded by two perfusionists plus assorted hangers- on. The exposures are wide and wonderful; you can stand at the OR table watching the heart pounding and pumping, the lungs inflating like bellows and the blood coursing in the big vessels as it turns from deep purple to brilliant scarlet. Then there's the well- choreographed drill of "going on bypass" and the dramatic uncertainty of "coming off", both spectacular hallmarks of these big operations, which have lots in common with high stakes sporting events. The whole show is really dramatic even if you've seen it a hundred times.

Neurosurgery, pretty much none of the above. Evolution has insured that the brain and spinal cord are encased in an almost continuous carapace of solid bone from skull to sacrum, so it requires a fair amount of ingenuity plus a good dose of hard work just to get a glimpse of either. Then after all that effort, the central nervous system just lays there, apparently not doing a damn thing. The brain, pale golden in color and wrinkled like an old man's face, is covered with a fine tracery of tiny pink arteries and larger blue veins. Its surface, the cerebral cortex, glistens because of the thin covering layer of cerebro-spinal fluid that's trapped against it by a spider-web-like membrane known appropriately as the arachnoid. The brain's major lobes clump together in a shape that roughly mimics a mushroom, with an irregular cap shrouding the stem; beneath the cap, a network of major nerves and vessels lay packed tight, encircling the stem in a complex anatomy lesson. Even under the brilliant illumination and stark magnification of the operating microscope, none of it appears very exciting. On close examination, the cortex moves gently with respiration and even more slightly with the heartbeat, but otherwise nothing. There are no clues; you have to come to this dance already knowing the steps.

On the other hand, if a young doctor is lucky or weird or perhaps just thoughtful, every time she sees the living brain, she's stunned again by the realization that these three pounds of protein and fat are the distilled essence of this unique individual, and that superficially, this clump of goo is a carbon copy of the mind /soul of every person that has ever lived. Insignificant as it appears to the naked eye, this organ is so important that the entire body is designed exclusively to protect, nourish, support, and transport it; to feed it information and do its bidding - at all costs. Nothing else truly matters. This *is* the person.

Breathtaking, because it's so undeniably true.

If a surgery intern who happens to wander through a neurosurgery operating room takes a look at the exposed brain and resonates with that emotion, even if just for a second, he or she is going to be a neurosurgeon. I first felt that way in late summer 1969, and it's still the way I feel every day. The bonus has been that I've loved everything that followed. Every year of involvement and learning has made the experience richer and more rewarding. And my sense of awe even greater.

Neurosurgery attracts young physicians like me because of the complexity of the central nervous system and the fascination of dealing with the essence of human existence. Within the specialty, some surgeons are drawn to the technical difficulties intrinsic in vascular and tumor surgery, some to the fascinating puzzles inherent in facilitation/inhibition of brain activity and others to correction of congenital defects in children. But whatever the choice, the stakes are extraordinarily high. These are bad diseases, and the system has a low level of tolerance for surgical error. Either way, the consequences for patients and families aren't a great recruiting tool, which is one reason young surgeons -in-training are required to spend countless hours in the ICU and its waiting room. That's where they learn about the downside of neurosurgery.

I've been very fortunate that the greatest advances in neurosurgery since its advent in the 1920s have all occurred within the relatively short span of my career. Almost exclusively they've been the direct results of dramatic, startling improvements in our ability to image the brain and spinal cord. Beginning with CT scanning in the early 1970s through the unbelievable refinements brought about by magnetic resonance imaging, neurosurgeons can now pinpoint structures as small as one millimeter anywhere deep within the brain's mass, which translates into more certain diagnosis pre-op, less damage going in, more precise work at the target and less collateral injury all around.

In 1970 it was common for even the best surgeons to operate for "something" – what was believed to be a tumor or an abscess or maybe a stroke- only to find absolutely nothing and to do serious damage in the process. For a competent surgeon, that's unheard of today. Pre-operatively, now he knows what "it" is, where "it" is, and generally the best route to go get "it". That in itself is so amazing it's difficult to imagine why a would-be surgeon would consider any other field, until you take into consideration that just as the brain is different than all other organ systems, afflictions of the central nervous system are unlike any other human diseases.

Because the brain IS, in fact, the patient- not just a component or a feature- diseases of the brain attack and often destroy the individual essence of a human being in a way other processes, some of which may be even more lethal, do not. For example, a patient's whose heart has been ruined by the ravages of atherosclerosis hasn't lost the unique ability to love, but one whose temporal lobes are injured may not even understand what that emotion is, nor be able to recognize those to whom it previously applied. Every volitional movement, sensory perception or behavioral emotion has its genesis in the central nervous system, which, despite its bony protection, is almost pathetically subject to injury and affliction. Unlike the cellular components of almost all of the body's other systems, the complex nerve cells of the brain and spinal cord are not capable of regeneration; when they're ruined they're done, and the neurosurgeon can't order a replacement thalamus from a catalogue or a substitute frontal lobe from a donor down the hall.

Fortunately, there is some plasticity and a little redundancy built into the nervous system, especially the very young nervous system. These two factors account for many of the "miracle" neurological recoveries that occur in some badly-injured neurosurgery patients. Although these "cures" don't happen frequently enough to completely overshadow the losses that characterize much of a neurosurgeon's practice, we're making a lot more of our patients well than was true forty years ago, and the promise of successful treatments for brain / spinal cord injury, tumors of the central nervous system and stokes is very bright- but still only a promise.

Said differently, these are still bad afflictions, often with heartbreakingly poor patient outcomes. In spite of all the new technical developments and bright therapeutic future, the practice of neurosurgery still has enough painful downside that the young surgeon really has to want to do this work. But if she does, it's the best job in the world, and a decision she'll never regret.

CHAPTER THREE

City Hospital (No.1)

SUMMER 1967

I was a rising junior at Washington University Medical School during the Summer of Love -1967- when the songs said everything was groovy, and everyone was going to San Francisco with flowers in their hair. It would have been a good time to be hanging out with my girlfriend down in Palo Alto, rather than smoldering in hot humid St. Louis where I was doing my first internal medicine rotation in a charity hospital that seemed like it was right out of the middle ages. Nah, I'm kidding; that's complete bullshit- I loved it.

City Hospital No.1 wasn't considered to be the armpit of medical care in town- that would have been City No.2, mostly for black people- but it was thought to be a close second, and as such, a proper spot for wet-behind-the-ears medical students to get a look at the seamy side of health care in the big city. There were a small number of real doctors somewhere in the hospital," real" meaning folks who'd finished their training and were earning a decent salary for what they did, but from my snake's-belly viewpoint I encountered only one in three months and I'll get to him later. With that significant exception, this poor man's health care circus was the sole property of the two residency training programs in town; all the boots on the ground belonged to docs in training, ranging from the lowest of the low junior medical students to

28

lordly senior residents who strode the halls in long, white lab coats, just one short year from being turned loose on the public.

Like most big city hospitals of that era, the wards were 'open', meaning huge rooms with fifteen to twenty beds down each of two walls, beds separated only by filthy cloth curtains which could be pulled together to enclose the individual beds for what passed as privacy. The wards themselves were designated by the presumed nature of the patients' diseases., or rather by the supposed appropriate treatment for those diseases; i.e. MEDICINE, SURGERY, OB, ORTHO, PEDS. If you as a patient were unlucky enough to have a MEDICINE disease and found yourself on a SURGERY ward, you might just get an operative procedure you didn't really need because: a) that was what they were serving; b) you were too dumb/drunk/coked-up to know the difference, or c) there weren't enough Spanish-speaking residents to sort out your symptoms. This was big-city indigent health care in 1967.

I spent my first six-week stint at CITY #1 as what was called an "extern", the most junior member of one of two teams on the Wash U MEDICINE ward. A "team" consisted of one junior resident, two interns and 2-3 externs (later known as sub-interns), junior medical students getting their first exposure to medicine in the raw. Above it all was one high and mighty "chief resident "who supervised both teams.

Generally each of the two teams on the service would "cover"- be responsible for- half of the ward's patients or about twenty folks with varying severities of illness. The teams alternated,one being "in the house" all night, every night, which meant mean we came in for rounds at 0600 on Monday, worked that day, that night and the next day until check-out rounds at about 1900 (7 PM) on Tuesday.

Each ward had three nurses (one R.N. and two L.V.N.s) from 7 AM to 3 PM and one LVN on the evening shift from 3PM to 11 PM. When that LVN left around midnight, there were two nurses' aides to take vital signs; otherwise, the teams were on their own, meaning that the "externs" passed all the medications, regulated the IV's, dealt with the myriad minor complaints of the patients and, starting about 5 AM, drew all the bloods and collected the urine samples for the morning labs.

According to the medical school curriculum, an extern's real job was to be furthering his/ her medical education. Ideally, the extern would be the first medical -type person to interview and examine each new patient, as well the first to respond to any issues with patients already on the ward. Again ideally, we'd take an extensive history of the patient's current illness, investigate the patient's past medical issues and medications, jot down their habits (remarkably, none had ever had more than two beers in a day), note their allergies, then haul out the stethoscope, otoscope, reflex hammer and sterile glove for a complete physical examination.

A good third year student could probably do the whole shooting match in an hour or so, given a cooperative patient, a quiet room, instruments that work, something to write with /on, and no interruptions. Then again ideally, the diligent med student would take his/her notes, retire to his/her call room, write up the findings, consider the potential most likely diagnoses, and then investigate those in his internal medicine text, in order to be ready to "present' that patient to his junior resident on command. The stated goal of the rotation was to repeat this process once every 'call day', which would mean that over a six-week time frame the student would "work up" around twenty patients, a good general introduction to the common internal medicine diseases which would ideally provide a strong foundation in interviewing and physical examination.

That process may have, in fact, happened somewhere, but not at City #1. The exigencies of the service being what they were, I actually did a complete history and physical on a grand total of six patients, exactly one a week. I had about thirty minutes every day to read about my patients, and I averaged six- to-seven hours sleep… out of every forty-eight. I did develop a nodding acquaintance with some parts of the physical examination: for instance, I could tell if the heart was actually beating and could recognize two of the most common arrhythmias (bigeminy and atrial fibrillation); I could percuss consolidation in a lung, actually hear some breath sounds and could feel a liver if it was really big. I learned what a thrombosed hemorrhoid looked like and could spot a big peri-rectal abscess every time. On the other hand, I never looked in any patient's fundi, couldn't find a spleen, missed at least four loud carotid bruits, one tracheal deviation and one enlarged thyroid. The one thing I did a lot of was rectal exams. The rules said there had to be one rectal exam on the chart for every patient; just by the nature of things it was always the extern's.

Speaking of the chart: By the end of the rotation, I could remember the proper order for recording the History and Physical without reference to my notes but my six formal work-ups never got anything higher than a C from our chief resident. One came back with the comment, "I think you're kind of pre- verbal." I missed every diagnosis but one; when the patient is bright yellow, liver failure is a pretty sure bet.

Contrary to what one might think, I loved this rotation. These were real people with real problems, things I understood viscerally if not yet intellectually, and by some magic I was actually part of a team trying to help them. Yeah, I couldn't hear a third heart sound, but by the end of six weeks I could have drawn blood from a turnip- no vein I couldn't hit, even if it took a couple of sticks. I didn't like passing meds much, but I could give you an intra-muscular injection of Keflin (which hurts like hell) and make you smile when it was over. I couldn't read EKGs worth a damn, but if we needed one done and the one tech in the hospital was busy and /or drunk (meaning always) I could whip a presentable strip out in reasonable time, even on an uncooperative patient in DTs.

More importantly, I got a glimpse of what medicine in the raw was like, what it could mean to sick people, and what it could cost its practitioners. The patients at City #1 were at the very bottom of America's health care pyramid; no social status, no money and not much hope. Often, regardless of whose fault it was, their lifestyles had made them "piss-poor protoplasm"; chronically undernourished, physically and psychologically neglected and emotionally unstable.

The young docs and would-be-docs at City #1 didn't start by asking, "How could this human mess happen? "but rather "How can we help?" and in an almost naïve, non-judgmental way, they busted their asses to make these societal outcasts what passed for healthy again. And admittedly, lots of these folks were sufficiently reprehensible as to make doing that difficult. As my chief resident would say more than once," We're not here to love them, just to get them well."

Having played some sports, I thought I knew a lot about team work, but at this big city hospital I saw it in a different context and learned a lesson that unfortunately remains a mystery to some of my generation and many in the generations that followed. The lesson goes like this: true teamwork is as much about caring for one another as about the team's stated mission. Being a part of and loyal to The Team was, and is, an incredible force that could keep you going when you'd had no sleep for two days, felt like dog shit and couldn't summon up one more ounce of compassion for the misery you saw around you. But you'd go the extra mile, if not for the patient, then because you couldn't let the Team down. Living that commitment even without fully understanding it would become even more important in my next six weeks, when I went downstairs to THE PIT.

Other than adapting to routine life in this new cultural jungle, one remarkable thing happened when I was "on the wards." Adjacent to MEDICINE 1 WARD was its surgery equivalent, also staffed by medical students, interns and residents from the two local medical schools. This was a primo rotation for the surgeons at every level because there was so much surgery to be done and no high-tone faculty members to "steal" cases. If you're operating for an average of thirty out of every forty-eight hours for six straight weeks, you can really rack up the cases. Surgeons learn by doing - that's what surgical education is all about. One of the lucky junior medical students doing a surgery externship on SURGERY ONE during my MEDICINE rotation next door was a housemate of mine; for the sake of this discussion, let's call him Larry Munn.

Larry was from Northern CA and my classmate in college although we hadn't known one another during those four years. He was a great guy, good jock, excellent student and maybe just a tad naïve. We shared the same on-call schedule, so while I was using a flashlight to peer up peoples' butts over in MEDICINE 1, he was scrubbing on big surgery cases, holding retractors and getting to sew up some of the monstrous incisions belly surgeons used back in 1967. Late in his rotation Larry honestly got to do most of an appendectomy skin-to-skin; consequently, he was the envy of everyone in the class. Naturally the silly SOB ultimately went into cardiology.

Larry and I were on call together one Saturday night when City #1 was balls-to-the-wall crazy. The ambulance sirens started about 5 PM and were steady until the sun staggered up late Sunday morning. On

MEDICINE 1 we caught eight direct admissions plus two folks we had to keep in the ER overnight for lack of beds. None of the six of us ever sat down; even the chief was working his butt off. Two of our long termers on the ward decided to die in the early morning, but not until we'd run full codes for what seemed like hours on each one. We were inundated by a tidal wave of sick folks; if you got admitted to City #1 that night you were what was called "low sick."

SURGERY 1 was just as busy; I knew because they had a couple of disasters among their ward patients and since both their teams were in the OR, we had to free up an intern and a scut-puppy (me) to jump into the middle of that chaos. Probably the biggest case they had going in the OR was the victim of one of the long running drug wars that were becoming endemic in the Midwest during the late 1960's. This particular hoodlum had in some way pissed off one of the reigning honchos. In response, he'd been shot several times while taking a dump in a PortaPotty outside a local bar. Don't ask me what a PortaPotty was doing in the bar's parking lot, other than the obvious. The police arrived to find the parking lot littered with fresh 9mm casings, so when the victim hit the PIT (ER), everyone knew Larry and his teammates were dealing with multiple 9mm. GSWs (gunshot wounds).

The nine-millimeter round was a new American fad. It would become the country's most popular hand gun round a decade or so later with the introduction of the new "plastic pistols "designed by Gaston Glock. The cartridge has a lot to be said for it: easy to shoot, minimal recoil, high magazine capacity, readily available here and abroad, etc. and it's sure as hell fatal if somebody in close proximity shoots you in the head. However, the Nine is not much of a manstopper, especially if the man in question is squatting (with the door closed) in a thick fiberglass PortaPotty, as was the case with Pedro, the patient that Larry's team caught about midnight on the evening in question.

In the PIT Pedro was bleeding like a stuck pig from eight GSWs scattered all over his skinny body; two in his chest, two in the belly, one in his butt (that must have been one hell of a shot) and the remainder in various extremities. By the time the police extricated him from his shattered fiberglass cocoon and got him to City #1, Pedro was shocky but still conscious and covered in feces. The surgery team took him straight up to the OR, giving him uncross-matched blood en route; once he appeared stable, the team hosed him down, shot a few x-rays and began to figure out from the calculated trajectories of the slugs what organs were supposedly at risk.

Bullets do crazy things; it's a well-known medical premise that when the target is a underworld denizen, it's likely that ballistic craziness results in "close, but no cigar." Larry's new patient- Pedro- again proved that old saw; he ended up with an exploratory laparotomy to oversew a stomach wound, a chest tube to re-inflate one lung and an open debridement of wounds to both hands and one foot. That's still 2 ½ hours of surgery time even though there was no need to crack Pedro's chest or open his head. After the general surgeons bowed out, the ENT guys took another hour or so to pick out all the fiberglass fragments from his face and mouth before sending him to the Recovery Room. There he got another unit of blood and was observed until he was conscious enough to start calling for pain medication and a lot of it. Recovery gave him 8 mg of morphine sulfate IM (a middling dose) and sent him down to SURGERY 1.

I was covering for Larry, and when I went into SURGERY 1 to check on the new arrival, the ward was in an uproar. Pedro was screaming at the top of his lungs and at least five other patients were cursing loudly in Spanish. Everyone else was wide awake, wondering what the hell was going on. Pedro calmed right down with a little more MS given IV, so I checked his vitals, adjusted his IV drip rate, gave his Foley catheter a look to make certain it wasn't crimped and told the ward nicely to shut up and go to sleep. The noise level dropped a little, not much, but I had other promises to keep, so after watching Pedro long enough to make sure the MS hadn't stopped his breathing, I headed back next door.

A couple hours later, I steamed out of MEDICINE headed for the PIT to check on one of our boarders and ran smack into a cluster of cops at the entrance to SURGERY 1. Two were the routine hospital security retirees, but the other three looked like serious business. I was giving them lots of room when I saw my buddy Larry in his bloody scrubs right in the middle of the scrum. Stopping to provide moral support, I noticed that the ward was absolutely silent; I could have heard a mouse (of which there was no shortage) fart. Once Larry ID'ed me for the cops, their attention shifted as they questioned me about when I'd put old Pedro to bed. Fortunately it was all in his chart. Unfortunately, his chart was hung on a hook at the end of his bed, where the privacy curtain was tightly drawn. There was a smattering of blood on the floor; as we walked over, no one spoke.

Larry was fresh out of the OR, having been dispatched by the powers that be to check on Pedro. He had known something was wrong when he found all the ward lights turned off and the ward itself completely silent. He'd located the light switch, flicked it on, seen the blood and ripped open the privacy curtain, certain Pedro was bleeding out from his stomach wound. His diagnosis was correct, at least in part. Pedro was bleeding out alright, but all his surgical wounds were clean and dry.

The police decided later that day that the guys who ventilated Pedro's PortaPotty must have shared my misgivings about 9mm. ammunition so they'd followed the ambulance that brought Pedro to City Hospital #1, then waited in the jampacked ER briefly before going upstairs to the operating room waiting area . Once Pedro was wheeled out of Recovery and onto the patient elevator, four men watched until the elevator reached the fifth floor, then waited patiently for the public elevator to take them to the same destination. How long they had to wait for Pedro to get moved into the ward bed, for me to respond to his shouts, medicate him and then go back to my own ward before they closed his curtain and almost cut off his head off is unknown, but I was grateful for their patience. Naturally, the 39 other patients denied seeing any late visitors, hearing anything unusual or knowing who extinguished the ward's lights. Before the cops left, one of them said, "Well, if at first you don't succeed …."

In every large hospital in which I've worked over the last forty years, the Emergency Room, Emergency Department, Emergency Whatever, has always been known by the folks who worked in the hospital as the PIT. That's in testimony to the raw, unfiltered aspect of human existence that's almost always on display just indoors from the ambulance dock and references a type behavior that affects /infects everyone that does business in the PIT.

I've been in some really nice PITs; brand new, spic and span, high tech and glistening. That was not the City Hospital #1 Emergency Ward. This PIT was old, dark and usually pretty dirty despite the best efforts of a heroic nursing staff and a genuine badass Medical Director I'll call Nathan Stern. He's the guy I mentioned previously who actually was a fully-trained physician in the employ of the hospital. He was the PIT BOSS.

Nathan, who everybody from the janitors to the head nurse called Nate, was late 30s, maybe 40; it was hard to tell and damn sure nobody was going to ask him. He stood about 5'5" in his black tennis shoes, probably went a buck twenty soaking wet, had black kinky hair and a face so badly ravaged by acne I thought he'd missed his small pox vaccination. He'd grown up somewhere in New York, although I came to believe he'd been whelped in a wolf's den. After being thrown out of more colleges than I'd had hot dinners, Nate had finally gotten in to one of the Caribbean medical schools, come back to Chicago for his internship and internal medicine residency and then worked in the ER at Cook County while looking for a private practice job in one of the suburbs out on the lake. That was a pipe dream; this guy was already a wild man and it only took one interview for any private hospital in its right mind to pass on that pending disaster.

After several years, apparently (meaning what people said behind his back) Nate's act was getting a little stale even at Cook County, so when the Metropolitan Health Department came looking for a medical director for City #1, all Nathan wanted to know was if he could live in the hospital. The Board was flummoxed by that one, but they compromised by leasing him an apartment in a pretty iffy building right across the boulevard from the hospital's ER entrance.

So early in July, Nate loaded everything he owned in a decrepit Dodge van for the move south. The Dodge cracked its block still within sight of downtown Chicago and consequently, the young doc was forced to get an advance on his first month's salary to buy a secondhand Ford pick-up and a tarp to cover all the stuff he had in the bed for the trip down south. At the used car lot, someone had to teach him how to work the truck's manual transmission before he launched on the Interstate. The story went that Nate still had junk left unpacked in the bed of the truck when the first snow fell in late November. No big deal, because from the moment he got to town, Nate basically lived in his hospital call room.

Just about this time (1967), hospital -based physicians and some nurses began to wear surgical scrubs on duty. This was a contentious issue for quite a while but ultimately everybody in the house adopted the dress, to the degree that now there are multiple designer scrub manufactures competing in what's become a lucrative national market. Ironically, Nate, the epitome of a rebel in many ways, was rabidly opposed to this cultural shift. If you worked in his ER as a doc (or a want-to-be-doc) you wore the traditional ice cream suit; white pants, short white coat, collared shirt and like it or not, a tie.

Meanwhile, nurses wore the traditional white nurses' uniforms and the old-style caps that designated the school from which they had graduated. If you've ever spent any time in a busy ER, you can understand that nurses wearing dresses can be a little problematic in terms of modesty, given some of the violent activities that are commonplace, but old Nathan was a genuine hard ass. It was his ball and his rules.

Nate got his laundry done free by the hospital, unlike the rest of us clowns, so every day he showed up in clean starched whites and one of several mangy-looking sport shirts that the laundry had done its best to destroy, but at least they were clean. What wasn't clean was the one tie he owned, which I would have sworn had been used to wrap fish. It didn't matter much because by about ten o'clock every morning the entire ensemble looked like a package of road kill. Nate could get more disgusting body fluids on him in a shorter time period than even the guys who worked in the morgue. The only thing that stayed clean on Nate was this big towel clip he wore clipped to his back pocket on the right. I thought it probably held his wallet in the pocket or something, but I was dead wrong. Fortunately I never had the balls to ask him.

This little squirt had a major league mouth; he could cuss like a West Texas roughneck, but he was an incredible doctor. Nate could smell a sick person from around the corner; he didn't have to examine them or inspect their labs or check their x-rays. A patient might look like a million bucks to everyone else but, if there was something wrong with the guy, Nate was on him like a hog on a snake and wouldn't turn loose until he found what it was. He could tell you what an EKG was going to show just by listening briefly to the chest, and watching a patient breathe for him was almost as good as a chest film. Naturally, Nate thought that the medical world outside "Internal Medicine- Emergency Medicine" was a bad joke. To him, surgeons were butchers, urologist plumbers, orthopedists mechanics, etc. This outlook made getting consultants to come to the PIT a little dicey, since the only ones that could stand the heat were a few old vets who had heard it all before and gave back just as good as they got. One general surgery chief resident's routine salutation when he came into the PIT was" Where is that little Jewish pissant?"

However, my favorite screw-Nathan line came from a senior Ortho resident who'd played offensive tackle at Missouri and was going back home to practice in Branson. Nathan had launched one of his typical tirades when the Orthopod put his big hand on the little guy's shoulder and said. "Nate, old buddy, where I come from you'd need to stand on a box to kiss my ass… and I'm not far from home." All well and good, but nobody had any problems with the way Nate took care of patients. He was also one of the most compassionate physicians I ever met.

If you put all of Nate's weirdness together, stirred an endless supply of really sick patients, a lot of young, true believer docs and then plopped that mess down in the pressure cooker of a big city ER, what bubbled to the top was charisma. Nate had it in spades.

Anyone who's ever worked in an ER or any acute hospital setting will testify that's it's almost impossible to render care to someone who's actively trying to resist, or even worse, to hurt you. Regardless of how small or weak the putative patient is, a single care-giver just can't be fighting off an assault with one hand and effectively rendering care with the other. The problem is obviously magnified if the person resisting is large, strong and hostile. Unfortunately, this is a problem ER personnel deal with on almost a daily basis; the rougher the clientele the bigger the issue. That's one of several reasons that most ERs have security details available but convincing someone to stop trying to kill you is different than having the person cooperate while you sew up his lacerations, examine her belly or check to determine if his/ her neck is broken.

The reasons people fight against receiving emergency medical care are multiple; fear, misunderstanding, and certain religious beliefs all at some time or another may play a role, as do mental illness like schizophrenia, paranoid delusional states and overt psychosis, but by far the most common cause is an altered mental state due either to drug or alcohol intoxication. It's hard to drum up much sympathy for a drunk who's just busted your lip simply because you were trying to clean a laceration on his ugly face, especially after he's vomited on your white coat, but almost always doctors and nurses manage to deal with these obstreperous individuals without any reciprocal hostility. However, the true violent bad actors pose a significant risk to people who are attempting to do nothing more than be of help. In some of these situations it's obvious the vodka or cocaine has unmasked a genuine sociopath.

In dealing with these latter assholes, physical restraints are worse than useless, there are never enough bodies to completely restrain the guy and the use of tranquillizing medications can be a little iffy until you really get to know something about the miscreant's medical condition, plus you've got to get an IV in the hostile patient first. Put it altogether and you've got a serious problem. Nate was an honors graduate of this course, all 120 pounds of him.

Nate never came into the PIT without this big towel clip snapped onto his back pocket. A towel clip is a ratcheted surgical instrument that looks like a large clamp or hemostat whose blades have been replaced by two curved very sharp pincers that meet in a fine point when the ratchet, which joins the two finger holes, is closed. Designed to pin surgical drapes or towels together and/ or to skin in the OR, towel clips are sufficiently strong, once they've been clamped onto bone, to test joints for stability. When truly sharp, the points make only a pinhole in skin. Nate's clip was needle sharp.

By far the biggest sensory nerve in the body is the trigeminal nerve that supplies sensation to the face, eyes, mouth, teeth, lips and importantly to the nose. This means that almost all forms of sensation to include pain are experienced with greater intensity in the distribution of the trigeminal nerve than elsewhere in or on the body. Just think about your own experience with bumping your lip, biting your tongue, or being whacked in the nose; almost insignificant trauma elsewhere on the body is magnified when the face is involved. One specific area where this sensitivity appears to be especially exaggerated is the columella of the nose, that pillar of skin and underlying cartilage at the tip of the nose separating the two nasal openings or nares. A little self-examination will prove that the cartilage here sits three or four millimeters below the surface skin of the columella, so there's a little room between the two tissues there, in fact just enough to accommodate the careful placement of the points of a sharp pincer.

The first time I heard about Nate's towel clip was during the week of the Major League Baseball All-star game in early July 1966, a time that corresponded with the worst heat wave the Mississippi Valley had experienced in the twentieth century. I saw the device in action the following summer, when the heat was almost as terrible. A major part of the hospital itself didn't have central air, so there were hundreds of window units trying to cool off the large wards, but the PIT and the ORs had some type of rudimentary central cooling that seemed to keep the temps in the low eighties. Outside it was miserable; temperature hovering around 100 and humidity about ninety during the days with minimal relief when the sun went down. The PIT was inundated with heat stroke victims, mostly the poor, the sick and the elderly. Taking care of just one heat stroke patient requires an enormous and continuous amount of human resources; taking care of a dozen at one time is a disaster.

Fortunately, early on in 1966, someone had learned that the only way to lower this number of folks' body temperatures to safe levels and then keep them there was to submerge the patients in ice baths. About thirty minutes after this discovery, the staff had three huge tubs set up in the PIT, each being filed with a combination of ice and water. The staff found that each tub would accommodate four to six patients and that every patient initially required the full-time attention of two care-givers, continually monitoring body temperatures, running IV fluids, watching urinary outputs, giving medications and trying to keep the patients conscious so they didn't slip down and drown in the slush. It was kind of a combination of water polo, tag team wrestling, and a rodeo; in 1967 it went on for 3 ½ days. The good guys won most but not all of the matches.

On the evening of the second day, which happened to be a Saturday, the local PD brought in two big drunk rednecks who had decided to take over a bar down by the river after someone objected to their uninvited massage of the female bartender. We were all busier than cats covering up shit on a tin roof with the heat strokes, but these bozos couldn't be ignored. Each of the tattooed rats went about 250, and neither could remember his last bath; they had no more than five healthy teeth between them. Their vocabularies were limited to "mutherfucka" and" I's gonna kill your ass", which made it pretty hard to take the classic medical history. Doing an actual physical exam was out of the question.

One of these gentlemen was handcuffed. For some reason the other was not, but with the cops' help, two of us grunts got them up on adjacent exam tables and focused the exam lights, so the nurses could begin cleaning up their battered faces. One of our student nurses was gently lavaging a forehead laceration on the cuffed guy when I heard him growl, "You stupid bitch!" That was punctuated by a hollow thump as he executed the first perfect head butt I'd ever seen. The nurse went down like she'd been beheaded. Just as the redneck was baring his two filthy teeth and looking around for new meat, Nate was on him like white on rice.

The little doc crawled right up on this shithead's chest, held the perp's head still with his left hand and out popped the towel clip. Deliberately, Nate snagged the columella, tugged just a little to free the skin from the underlying cartilage, and as the ratchet closed I could hear the clicks across the room. Nate looked the guy right in the eye, tugged on the handles and said, "Now you sorry son-of-a-bitch -shut up and be still".

The red neck looked like he'd been struck by lightning and stopped breathing. I was hoping for a full blown respiratory arrest, mainly because he deserved it but also because I hadn't gotten to intubate anybody yet, but in about 20 seconds he took a very shaky breath and said in a shivering voice, "Y-Y-Yes sir."

Nate climbed down from his chest, looked around and handed the towel clip to me. He said, "I think we've got his attention," then went to check on the student nurse, who was going to have a huge bruise on her forehead and a great story to tell her classmates. It got even better when, once we'd cleaned this dirt ball up, it was obvious he had a suture-able laceration in his scalp just above his right ear. I got to sew up the lac (my first)and guess who got to hold the towel clip? She did a great job- only tugged on it a couple of times, maybe once extra just for luck.

In the summer of '67, if you were young, hungry and didn't mind a little road rash, forget the flowers in your hair. City Hospital #1 was the place to be.

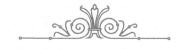

CHAPTER FOUR

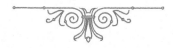

Two Men

As a part of my six-year post-graduate program (internship and residency) there was a consecutive twelve months period labeled "elective", during which I could pursue any aspect of neurology or neurosurgery that I could convince my chairman was even potentially germane to my education. As a rule, most of my cohorts elected to do some basic neurology, and because we weren't limited to our own institution, many of them went to London to the neurology course at the historically famed Queen's Square Hospital for Diseases of the Nervous System. Along with its French equivalent La Pitie, Queen's Square is one of the most famous neurology -neurosurgery institutions in the free world. These two renowned hospitals have been the sites of many of the important developments in the two specialties over the last two centuries. Naturally I passed on that opportunity.

Instead, because I'd spent seven months in France as a college student and still spoke some very marginal French, I wanted to spend my elective year working in a different French hospital for a French neurosurgeon named Gerard Guiot. Professor Guiot, who was in the process of re-inventing the basic concepts of pituitary surgery, spoke excellent English and was known to be a fan of young American neurosurgeons. In addition, during my third year of training he was making a serendipitous stop in Dallas to give a couple of lectures. The stars were aligned.

I cleared the proposed project with my chairman and then during Professor Guiot's visit, my wife at that time (who spoke fluent French) and I invited the visitor over for an aperitif. After the first glass of wine, we pitched the deal right there. Even though we came at him out of left field, Guiot was the epitome of graciousness and agreed that we could probably work something out. Ultimately, with his help we cleared all the regulatory hurdles, and the professor secured a grant (called a *bourse*- the French word for purse) to finance my year's stay on his service. The grant came from the French Ministry of Foreign Affairs and was usually reserved for visiting physicians from medically underdeveloped countries, so this was an impressive display of Guiot's standing in France, and as the year wore on, it got even more impressive.

My wife, during her year as a college exchange student at the Sorbonne, had become friends with an elderly lady who owned an apartment located in Paris' 16th arrondisment. This beautiful district is fortuitously situated just across the famous Bois De Boulogne from Guiot's hospital in the small town of Surenes. The Bois, a huge park and the historic hunting ground of the French kings prior to the revolution of the 1770s, was only two city blocks from Senora Feliciana Lopez' apartment. This lovely lady, one of the kindest people I've had the pleasure to know, offered to lease us the servant's quarters of her apartment for the length of our stay.

Once we got moved in and figured out the local landscape I took off across the Bois to Surenes to meet with Dr. Guiot and his team. After listening to me struggle through rounds with my marginal French, the chief resident (chef des residents) took me in tow, introduced me around and then as a parting shot, made it clear that I, as a member of the *equipe,* was invited to the wedding of one of the junior residents the following Saturday. I lied, saying I'd love to come, but might need a little help in finding the church. He smiled and said, "Probably not." The kid was getting married in Notre Dame.

So, on Saturday at the appointed hour I showed up at the cathedral's front doors. When I didn't recognize anybody on the portico, I sneaked inside, figuring I'd have to check all the side chapels for the ceremony, but no way. The main sanctuary was almost completely full. It turned out the bride's father owned most of the appliance stores from Chartres to the Belgian border. I spotted the Foch residents, then worked my way over to stand next to the Chef. He welcomed me with a handshake and a big hug, then went back to paying attention to the ceremony.

Toward the end of the homily, I looked around for Professor Guiot without any luck. It was hard to believe he'd miss this event, but as the recessional began to boom from the great organ I still couldn't locate my soon-to-be mentor, so I whispered my question in Chef's ear. He turned with a huge smile on his face, pointing up and behind us at the organ, which was now playing at full volume. "That's the boss!" I'd later learn that Dr. Guiot was routinely invited to substitute for the cathedral's principal organist.

Hospital Foch, named for the French hero of the First World War, was part of the University Hospital system in Paris. An old but not antiquated facility, it catered primarily to so-called "private" neurosurgery and plastic surgery patients referred either to Professor Guiot's unit or to the service of Professor Paul Tessier, a magician of a plastic surgeon who was personally creating the specialty of cranio-facial malformation surgery.

Tessier was not only the reigning king of plastic surgery in Europe, but also was the current darling of French society. He was on radio, TV, and at every gala worth the name. If you were a wealthy Parisienne in the 1970s and needed your face lifted, your boobs made bigger/smaller, or your nose chiseled, Professor Tessier was the man of the moment. He did that kind of work two days a week at his private surgical clinic near the Arc de Triomphe, then came to Foch on the other two days to disassemble and reconstruct children's misshapen heads. Not only that, but since a lot of these kids were destitute North Africans, many times he paid to fly them to Paris, convinced the government to subsidize their medical bills, then flew them back on his own nickel to Algeria. He personally also paid the bills for the parents' travel and accommodations. Professor Paul Tessier was a serious player.

Professor Guiot and his number two, Patrick Derome, worked with Tessier on most of these kids, so I had a chance to watch this magic up close. The contrast between the "before" and the "after" was stunning.

Even more amazing were the actual surgical procedures themselves, when one plastics team would be completely dismantling the child's skull while the neurosurgeons were busy keeping the brain out of harm's way and the second plastics team would be removing every other rib from both sides of the kid's chest to use in reconstructing the head.

After 10-12 hours, they'd bandage the child up and wheel him into the special ICU, where the critical care specialists (called "re-animateurs") would take over, and I do mean take over. Us surgical types were only allowed to come in once each day, and then only to change dressings; we couldn't write any orders, change any medications or even touch the drains, tubes or ventilators. After ten days to two weeks, when we'd finally remove all the dressings, I literally couldn't recognize the children. Except for the inevitable bruising they looked like normal kids, and their parents would be dumbstruck. Truly inspirational surgery done by three incredible men.

When Professor Guiot wasn't helping with this kind of case, he was busy operating a variety of routine spinal problems, brain tumors and his specialty, tumors of the pituitary gland. He, along with one of his teachers, the English surgeon Norman Dott, had resuscitated an idea from the 1880s about approaching pituitary tumors, not through an incision on the head, but by an exposure up through the patient's nose and sinuses. Using the new operative microscope and very fine instruments Guiot often could not only remove tumor with essentially no trauma to the surrounding brain, but also spare what remained of the normal pituitary gland. Nobody in the States had caught on to this trick as of yet, although in another ten years almost all pituitary tumors throughout the world would be removed in this fashion, so it was a good and not terribly complicated technique to learn and ultimately bring back home.

Gerard Guiot himself was a true Renaissance man. A classical musician, a pen-and-ink artist and a master neuro-anatomist, he was a devout Catholic and a passionate French patriot. His mentor and father figure, Clovis Vincent, had committed suicide in protest when the Nazis entered Paris in 1940, and Guiot himself had spent the war as an expatriate surgeon working in a London hospital, but he was a "new European", a Frenchman who lectured often in Germany and was more than willing to accept young German neurosurgeons for training.

The professor routinely prayed with his patients prior to surgery in the most unassuming and natural fashion possible, and was incapable of harsh or bitter speech, which worked to his detriment in the cutthroat world of French academic medicine. His trainees swore by him and he was godfather to more children than he could count. Professor Guiot's wife was an associate curator of Egyptian antiquities at the Louvre; together they were the type people that give intellectualism a good name. He was also the best classical neurosurgeon I ever saw operate, either in the spine or in the head.

In 1972, Professor Guiot was operating about 140 pituitary tumors a year, usually three to four a week when he wasn't on the road giving talks, so there were lots of learning opportunities for a young guy like me. Then suddenly one Monday, after I'd been on the service about five months, there were none. During the weekend the Professor had been at his country farm when he developed chest pain and shortness of breath. By the time he'd arrived back at Foch, he'd suffered a major myocardial infarction. After the initial week, when the hospital grapevine told us the cardiologists were pretty sure he was going to live, everyone on the team looked around and realized there were no more pituitary patients. The extensive referral network Guiot had built over twenty years had dried up completely, and his two ORs stayed essentially empty for months.

I was sharing the two cranio-facial cases each week with two other visiting fellows, so now there was a lot of free time to spend contemplating my navel and thinking about how my last six months in Europe were going to be a complete waste of time. There is an unattractive selfishness and /or impatience that sometimes affects young, ambitious people when their plans are unexpectedly derailed, and to my discredit I had it bad. This despite my affection for Guiot and my relief that he was recovering well and probably would be able to return to practice after some six month's convalescence. Meanwhile I would be spinning my professional wheels and feeling sorry for myself right up to the moment I got back on the plane to Dallas. Pitiful, but true.

So, during one of my visits with Guiot- who was still in his ICU bed-he asked me how the service was going. Now, he knew exactly how the service was going; what he wanted to know was how I was doing in his absence. He's sixty-three, just survived a major MI, not healthy enough to be released from the ICU and he's concerned about how this thirty-one year- old student he's paying to live in Paris is getting along. So, I told him things were pretty slow and that I would be long gone before he came back to practice. He said he was very sorry, that maybe I could find a project to do in the lab, etc. When I didn't jump all over that idea, he asked if I knew of any other possibilities, and after a second, I admitted I did.

A friend from my own residency program, Dr. Larry Rogers, had recently finished his six months at Queen's Square and had taken ten days to visit two other neurosurgery programs in Europe. On his way home, he'd stopped to spend the night with us in Paris, and during an all-nighter over several bottles of wine, he'd told me about his life-altering experience in Zurich Switzerland.

For a couple of years, there'd been rumors of a new, hotshot neurosurgeon operating at the University of Zurich who, it was universally agreed, was a genuine horse's ass but supposedly an amazing surgical technician. My friend, Larry, who was (and still is) a pretty significant horse's ass himself, had decided to go have a look. He told me that what he'd seen in three days in this guy's OR was nothing less than the future of neurosurgery, and that it would be a lot less painful for me to learn it from the source than from his own amateur interpretation. But, he said, "You're damn sure going to have to learn it somewhere, because this is the real deal."

This new star's name was Mahmud Gazi Yasargil. Turkish, by birth, he'd gone to medical school as a kid in Nazi Germany during the last days of WW ll, then come to Switzerland for his general surgery, pathology, neuro-radiology and finally his neurosurgical training. He was forty-eight years old, and had spent a year recently at the University of Vermont; he spoke excellent English, in addition to Turkish, German, a little French and Switzer-Deutsch, the Germanic dialect spoken in about half of Switzerland. He was the number two guy in the neurosurgery department in Zurich where the chief, a native-born Swiss named Hugo Krayenbuhl, was due to retire in months. Yasargil had apparently made it clear he was leaving if he didn't get the head job, but the medical school had never had a non-native born Swiss as a department chair. Kind of a dicey deal to jump into, but I was out of other options.

So, I told Professor Guiot what I'd heard about Yasargil and that I'd like to leave his service to see what was what over in Zurich. He listened carefully, then told me he'd heard very good things about this new guy and that on the couple of times they'd met, Dr. Guiot had been impressed. So then, with me still sitting there, he calls down to his office, gets Yasargil's number and has the ICU ward clerk get the man himself on the phone. I can only hear one side of the conversation, which is in English, but it's all good news and in five minutes, I've been accepted for a six-month's stay in Zurich. As if that wasn't enough, after Dr. Guiot hangs up, he calls his secretary again for the number of the French Ministry of Foreign Affairs, then in a slightly longer conversation, convinces some bureaucrat to let this American take his French money to Switzerland. Not exactly the anticipated response.

The only rational explanation for Dr. Guiot's behavior was that he was overanxious to be rid of me. In fact, evidence suggests that wasn't the case. He made my exit from Foch painless, called Yasargil a couple of times to check on me and then, when we came through Paris headed back home, arranged a small dinner party at his apartment for us and the team members. I remain grateful for and embarrassed by his consideration and kindness. M.G. Yasargil was a different experience.

I arrived in Zurich in early March. Fortunately, we found an apartment in the nearby suburb of Zollickerberg, adjacent to a large, well-manicured forest-like park, which became critical for my sanity later on. The department of neurosurgery had sent me an introductory letter, telling me where and when to appear, so at 0800 hours on a Monday I show up at the door to the department's offices 'raring to go'. I spend about an hour with Yasargil's secretary, a Fraulein Trauber, doing the usual paper work, most of which is explaining how I'm going to support myself during this six-month period (the Swiss didn't want their landscape littered with itinerant, insolvent medical trainees).

This verification actually entailed a phone call back to Paris just to insure I hadn't forged the *bourse* contract. During the call it becomes obvious the French are just as confused by the situation as Trauber, but they all finally agree I'm legit. Fraulein Trauber decides I'm good to go and summons an orderly (Hans) to get me suited up and down to where Dr. Yasargil is doing his magic. Naturally Hans doesn't speak English, French or Spanish, so we grunt at one another and I get a large-grand-gross set of scrubs, change in the washroom and down we go.

Protocol in every OR is unique to that locale, so I don't think much of it when Hans walks me up to this huge metal barn-like sliding door, raps once sharply then rolls the door open and urges me to enter. I've taken two steps into the room before I realize someone has completely screwed the pooch. The super- sized OR is as silent as a tomb, and everyone-meaning the surgeon who I assume is The Man himself, his assistant, the scrub and circulating nurses, two anesthesiologists and the five guys sitting on steel stools up against the wall- are all staring at me. Hans rolls the door shut. I can't hear him giggling but I know the son-of-a-bitch is. After about 15 seconds, I say very softly; "Duke Samson, from Dr. Guiot."

The surgeon points his scalpel at me and with an absence of enthusiasm, says: "Shut up and sit down." There are a couple of empty stools, so very quietly I make my way over to take a seat. He watches me until I'm still, then turns back around, mutters something that makes the scrub nurse giggle and goes back to operating. I take a deep breath, but the misery is not quite over. I don't have a clue what he's doing- is this a tumor or an aneurysm or what? The guys beside me are acting like I've got some communicable disease, but I can see the x-rays are on a view-box over by the door I just stumbled through, so I get up to have a look.

"Sit down-sit down- SIT DOWN!" Now he sounds like he's really pissed, or at least if I sounded like that I'd be really, really pissed. I've been here a grand total of about ten minutes and can tell I've already ruined the next six months. Hunched on my stool, I'm wondering if Guiot will take me back, when Yasargil and his assistant step away from the table so the circulating nurse and an attendant whose name I'll learn is something like Guppy, wheel in the operating microscope. This thing is a monster. It's big enough to ride and has arms and attachments I don't recognize, but the most important thing it has is a giant camera that transmits what the surgeon is seeing to the two video monitors in the room. Once they turn on its lights I'm like Alice in Wonderland.

It's a physical impossibility to go without oxygen for thirty minutes, which is about how long it took Yasargil to take out this little brain tumor, but I would have sworn I didn't breathe once during the entire procedure. The technology that allowed me to see what he was doing was amazing in itself, but the guy's skill was jaw-dropping, even for a neophyte like me. He operated like he was born doing it and made it look so natural that I could even imagine myself making the same moves. It was the best movie I'd ever seen.

After he'd gotten the tumor out, he pointed his bayonet forceps at a structure, then turned to look at me. "You, Guiot's boy- what's that?"

If he thought I hadn't been paying attention he just didn't understand my fascination with the brain and the way he was displaying it, so I said, with real enthusiasm: "That, sir, is the pituitary stalk." Snort. "And what's that?"

"Right internal carotid artery, sir." "And this here?"

"I think that's the Membrane of Lillequist, Professor Yasargil."

"Correct. But "professor" is Herr Dr. Krayenbuhl. Don't call [me] Professor …. yet." He looked up at his scrub nurse. "Is good boy." She nodded, and I could tell she was smiling … at me.

I thought, "Holy shit. This is my kind of place."

In the daily journal I kept faithfully throughout my time in Zurich, it quickly became too tedious to write Yasargil's name every time I thought it necessary, so early on I adopted the abbreviation "YSG", and for old times' sake I'll follow that habit in in describing that fantastic experience now 45 years later.

I stayed in Zurich almost seven months and only left when I was dead broke and absolutely had to go back to Dallas. It was unbelievably good. I'd been there a week when the powers that be did the right thing and made YSG the chief. Apparently, he'd been so hard to get along with that all the Swiss residents were openly lobbing for him to not get the job, so the day after the announcement was made he lowered the hammer. YSG couldn't actually fire them but he basically banished them from his OR, and guess who was left to be his assistant? One week in town and I'm first-assisting the brightest rising star in world neurosurgery on every case. As I said, "Holy Shit!"

Many of the operative procedures YSG was doing in 1973 would still be tours de force today, but back then they were pure technical miracles. His approaches were all based on an encyclopedic knowledge of the brain's anatomy and he'd literally written the textbook about the brain's blood vessels. He'd developed and honed his microscopic technique doing countless practice procedures in the animal laboratory, read everything that had ever been written about intra-cranial neurosurgery, and... he had the balls of a cat burglar. He knew when he could go fast, and then he was faster than anyone else. When he started going slowly you knew he was defusing a horrible booby trap or dodging a fatal ambush. Whereas a very accomplished neurosurgeon could feasibly get two large cases done between 8 in the morning and 4 in the afternoon, YSG could do four, put in every stitch himself, be done by 2 P.M. and looking around for something else to do for the rest of the day.

I'd stand there beside him, occasionally lending a hand but usually more audience than assistant, watching like a hawk as he'd blaze through the day's "list" with effortless speed. For the first two weeks I never said more than "Yes sir" and "No sir" except to answer a direct question. YSG wasn't interested in conversation, music or anything other than doing the operation in front of him. The OR was absolutely silent; he had lots of visitors and routinely threw them out for talking, walking, coughing or for wrong answers to his questions. This wasn't a collegial atmosphere, but more like a royal audience.

He was an absolute monarch and you were there to observe, nod applause and finally to worship. If you didn't like it, just hit the road, Jack. He'd tell the next platoon of visitors what a turd you were.

YSG was capricious, petty, flammable, vindictive and a bully. Most importantly, he was a genuine genius inventing masterpieces that saved patients' lives by the hundreds in the 1970s and by the millions as his techniques spread across the civilized world. And by sheer luck, I was there at the creation.

At the end of the surgical day, he'd scurry off to see new patients or work on editing his operative videos, and I'd trudge down to the animal lab, where a congenial young Swiss technician I knew as Herr Luedtke would have an operative site set up for me and a white rat already anesthetized and prepped. There, under a rudimentary microscope, I'd do every dissection exercise that the Professor had invented, everything from exposing each and every abdominal organ, transplanting kidneys, sewing vessels together. At first, I'd use short instruments and then later on I'd work through a plastic yogurt cup with the bottom removed positioned over my "patient" to force me to use longer, bayonetted tools. Occasionally there would be another Zurich resident there briefly or a visitor would drop in to try his hand, but generally it was just Herr Luedtke, me and my "patients", the rats.

From time to time, I would sense an unannounced presence behind me, and looking up, I'd find the Professor inspecting my work. He'd watch, grunt and leave- no conversation, critique or suggestions. By that time of day, I'd usually had about all of YSG that I could take, so no big deal.

Around five in the afternoon, I'd clean up, take the tram out to Zollickerberg, say hello to my wife then change clothes and go running in the park to blow my head clean. Make no mistake-YSG was a giant pain in the ass to work around. For the entire day the tension in his OR was palpable even when he didn't go up in smoke. After walking that tightrope, a couple of hours in the lab trying to make my clumsy fingers imitate his effortless moves sewing 1 mm. arteries together with suture the width of human hair would leave me feeling ready to explode. After a week of coming home and railing at my wife, I realized that putting thirty minutes to an hour in on the park's roads was going to be mandatory if we were going to live through this time.

YSG hated the days when he'd be ready to start his first case but there weren't any visitors to gape at whatever miracles he was set to perform that morning. He'd grump to me: "What, don't they want to learn?" And even though he really disliked starting late, if a visitor would show up as I had in the mid- morning, Fraulein Trauber would call down to the OR and the Professor would delay his start until he had an audience. Ironically, he would treat that person like a visiting fireman, even if he was just some itinerant neurosurgery resident like me. The man loved an audience.

On a Thursday, right at the end of my stay, my last French check arrived, and just in time because we were dead broke, and the week-end was almost here. So, the next morning, a Friday, I would have to make it to the bank to cash the check during business hours, which meant I was not going to be available to assist YSG in the OR. The day before, I cautiously explained my problem to the Professor who first told me what a great case I was going to miss, and then growled that it would be OK. By that time, he'd told the Swiss residents they'd better get with the program or find another job so there were other alternatives to assist him.

I'm standing at the door when the bank opens, and for once there are no problems cashing the check, then changing French francs into Swiss ones, so I'm back at the Kantonsspital lickety split. Once I get suited up, I step very quietly into the small anteroom that has a viewing window into the OR- what I see ain't good. First, YSG is already in a tirade about something; the windows are sound proof, but no question he's having a major hissy. Second, there are no-zero- visitors. Five steel stools lined up in a row against the wall behind him are completely empty. This is an explosive situation, especially before the case really gets underway, and I'm thinking about re-visiting the bank, when Sister Dianne (YSG's scrub nurse and subsequent wife) sees me in the window. She bends down to speak to the Professor who whirls around, gesturing for me to get my sorry ass in there. I salute and head for the door.

He treats me like visiting royalty and is elated when I tell him I already know what the case is and am SO glad I got back in time to watch. That was no lie; he was doing an unusual opening which I figured I'd never get another chance to see before I had to do one on my own, but there was a problem. Sitting on these stools behind the surgeon's back, it was very difficult to see what was going on before the microscope was brought into the field, and that first part of the operation- the opening- was the very part of the case I needed to see. He doesn't let anyone ever get up from the stools and I'm not willing to push my luck even at this late date, but I figure if I slide over to the stool at the very end of the row and lean way out I can probably visualize most of what's going on.

So long story short, he's operating like mad and I'm stretched out to the limit trying to watch, when the stool slips out from under me. I fall flat on my large ass and all five stools do a slow-motion domino number.

It's by far the most noise for the longest time I've ever heard in an OR; in retrospect I'm surprised the patient didn't awake from anesthesia.

So, there I am sprawled on the floor, the stools are still clattering; YSG spins around with the scalpel in his hand, reaches out to me and says…" Are you O.K.?"

Sister Dianne cracks up and pretty soon everyone is laughing, probably because they were certain he was going to cut my throat. Once I got off the floor, he made me stand right behind him and explained every move of his opening. That day, I didn't go to the park.

During my thirteen months in Europe, I met two of the giants of my profession, two very different men. Gerard Guiot was a gentleman, a humanitarian, a compassionate teacher and a caring physician. He was the best classical neurosurgeon I've had the privilege to watch operate. Gazi Yasargil is a petulant prima donna, a volatile surgeon and a terrible teacher. To be honest, I think hidden in there somewhere is probably a compassionate individual but his incredible, consuming need for acclaim and applause have obscured that person from most of even his greatest admirers, of whom I'm definitely one. He is also the single most important surgeon in the two-hundred-year history of neurological surgery; the man who I believe has made more quantum leaps in advancing the craft of surgery that any comparable individual. He will be remembered, and honored, by the perpetuation of his ideas for as long as we have human surgeons operating on human brains.

It's of note that my buddy, Dr. Larry Rogers, who got me involved in this entire goat rope, has recently published a beautiful in-depth biography of this complex, amazing surgeon entitled simply "Yasargil". You can find it online.

CHAPTER FIVE

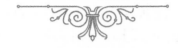

Trouble

The two of us were hanging out in the call room, watching a replay of a Texas high school football game and drinking stale coffee filched from the nurses' station when both of our pagers went off. Richard looked over at me.

Older, wiser and in charge, I didn't even flinch as I squelched the squawk. "All yours, Ace. I'm just here for the entertainment and refreshments."

"Right; don't move a muscle. Let your over-worked junior resident do all the work." Richard picked up the house phone and jabbed the key pad without muting his pager. Still watching the high schoolers knock each other out, he muttered, "Yeah, this is Neurosurgery- whatcha got?"

He listened, then sat up straight. "Be right there- don't move her." He dropped the receiver into the cradle.

"Need to go boss. They've got a pregnant girl down in the PIT that sounds like she's trying to die. Some kind of spinal cord thing they think. She's not moving her arms or legs and just stopped breathing while she's looking at them. Want to sit on your large ass here while I check it out?"

He was down the hall and on the stairs before I could get the tube turned off and shrug into my lab coat. As I was going through the door the pager squawked again, this time with the 911 code. I thought," The ER has its panties in a wad on this one," and headed for the elevator bank.

Metropolitan Memorial Hospital is a huge and justifiably famous trauma center. In testimony to the nature and volume of misery it draws, during the 1970s more than 100 GSWs of the head regularly made it past the Triage Desk and into the Surgery ER...every year. STAT calls here were a daily occurrence; multiple STAT calls meant somebody thought the shit was definitely in the fan.

By the time my elevator had made it down seven flights and I'd wended my way through the routine chaos outside the PIT, my pager was squawking 911 again. I turned the damn thing off, nodding at the two cops stationed at the double doors to the Surgery portion of the ER. When the doors swung open I dodged a lab tech and a frazzled medical student in a short white intern's jacket soaked with blood who looked at me, then pointed over his shoulder to the Trauma Hall. "She's in Trauma Two – you better hurry."

Every metropolitan hospital has a trauma hall-equivalent; two to four big, bright, fully-equipped operating-type rooms where the ER docs, surgeons, nurses and their helpers make medicine's last stand on behalf of the wounded from the big city's streets. When you add in the families and assorted morbidly-curious hangers-on, the scene looks and sounds like Texas Chainsaw Massacre at midnight on Bourbon Street.

I shouldered open the big door to Trauma 2, knocking down a radiology tech student in the process. My buddy Richard was center stage, crouched over the head of a thin form laid out on a very short OR table under one of the heavy ER lights. The second light was suspended over four guys in OB scrub suits down at the other end and I realized the patient was up in GYN stirrups. Blood pooled on the floor and the OB guys radiated an intensity that meant a real catastrophe was unfolding.

I helped the tech up, muttered my apologies and detoured around the OB contingent to come up beside my junior resident. He held the young woman's head between his hands, looking as if he was trying to pull it off her slender neck.

"Duke, those fucking clowns are going to kill her, the way they're working her butt back and forth down there. She's already a pretty high quad and I can't keep her neck straight when they're torqueing her around. Can't you stop them?"

On of the many advantages of doing a long residency- say six years- in one hospital is that toward its end, you've come to know most of the players in the system. Gary Buckingham, the big guy in charge of the action down at the table's other end, was in his final year of OB-GYN training. Smart as a whip with a mouth to match, Dr. Buckingham would be coming back to join the faculty after doing a two-year stint with the Air Force. Big as all outdoors, he also was one hell of a rugby prop. I'd spent many Sunday afternoons with my head lodged against his broad butt in the Dallas Ramblers rugby scrum.

"Gar, you knuckleheads cut that shit out down there. This woman's spinal cord is getting twisted around like a wet noodle."

'Listen asshole- if we don't get this baby out ASAP we'll have two dead bodies. The kid is in severe distress, not moving and..."

"Well, goddamn it, cut her open and deliver the damn thing before we lose them both. You don't need anesthesia- as far as we can tell she's completely out below the clavicles- so just do it."

Pause. "Christ, you're right." Over his shoulder he said," Open the section tray and get us a couple of suctions."

Two of the OB team backed away as he poured iodine prep over the swollen belly while one of his residents grounded the patient to the Bovie. Then the OB doc stuck hands that looked like meat hooks into a pair of size nine surgical gloves.

I'd seen all the C-sections I ever wanted to see, so I turned back to help Richard stabilize the sweat- stained head. "You're sure she's out, right? No sensation?"

"You bet."

And sure enough, the woman never twitched as Gary and his crew opened the belly and popped the fetus out in what seemed like seconds. For a minute there was amniotic fluid and blood everywhere, provoking Richard to snap at one of the ER nurses," Start that second unit of red cells and get us some more. Once they get done, I think we're going upstairs." The ORs were on the second deck, and pretty much a sure bet for this patient.

I didn't even want to look at the controlled chaos down south, but in a moment, we heard a faint squeak and Dr. Buckingham was holding up the tiniest baby I'd ever seen. "I think we've got a keeper. Pretty small, probably six weeks early, but she looks OK for a preemie."

"Nice work, fat man. Now clean that mess up and get the hell out of here so we can figure out what's what with Mom."

He put the baby in the incubator, shot me the bird and told his troops to get started closing ASAP. Nice to be working with a professional.

It took about another 90 minutes to give the girl three units of red cells and get a half-assed myelogram which showed that her problem to be a large, swollen something about six centimeters in length right in the middle of her cervical spinal cord. Although the images weren't good enough to identify the mass, without any history of trauma, the odds were high that the hemodynamic stresses of pregnancy had caused the rupture of a small birthmark-like blood vessel abnormality in the cord itself. The clot that I guessed was there but couldn't see on the myelo had probably grown big enough to put pressure on the cord around it to the degree that it simply stopped working. Whatever that damn thing was, for certain the cord wouldn't function again as long as it looked like that. Whether the swollen spinal cord had the capacity to do its duty once the mass was gone was anybody's guess. Richard and I sure as hell didn't know.

"So, here's the deal, junior. Either we leave her like she is- which means she'll never be able to breathe without a respirator or do anything more than shrug her shoulders, or else we go get that mystery out of there and take the pressure off the cord. If the operation doesn't kill her, she might have a shot. Whatta you think?"

He looked at me like I was nuts. "No chance versus maybe some chance – right? She's 34 years old, has two other kids. It's not even a question."

"Yeah, pretty much the way I see it as well, but... there's no way we can ask her with all the meds she's got on board, that tube jammed down her throat, and her paralyzed from the neck down. What's the story with her family? Where's the husband?"

"The OB guys said the family doesn't speak any English, and the husband is in prison. One of the translators told Gary that the guy's in for manslaughter, so we won't be seeing him this evening. Her mother is next of kin, and that's another problem, as if we needed one."

"Lay it on me."

"Mom's a Jehovah's Witness, so we've already pretty much screwed the pooch there. I don't know where we go to get permission to operate on her."

I shook my head; I'd taken care of lots of Witnesses. "There's more slack in that system than you think. Our lady has gotten some blood, sure, but the thing is, I'll be she didn't give anybody permission to transfuse her. We did it without asking, which as far as the Witnesses are concerned means she's off the karma hook- not her fault. Going forward, if they say "no blood" we've got to respect that, but I think we can get in and out of her neck without much blood loss, unless that mass is some bloody tumor or bad AVM, which ought to show up on the CT. Anyhow, I'm probably going to cheat and give her one more unit while we're waiting. Let's find that translator lady and talk to Grandmother."

We operated on Maria Elena Sanchez for a little more than four hours. Through a long incision extending from her hairline to the end of her neck, we separated the slender muscles of the spinal column then drilled away the bony roof of the canal and opened the parchment-like dura matter to expose the cord itself. Normally a tubular structure, cream colored and a little less than an inch wide, Maria's spinal cord was grossly swollen, pale white and distorted like a python that had eaten a pig. It humped up out of our bony opening, and when I spilt it open in the midline with a diamond knife, a thick cheesy fluid oozed out to fill the gutters of the canal.

"Shit- it's pus.' Richard looked up at me from the observer's scope. "The spinal cord is full of pus. That's the worst thing I've ever seen."

"Not so sure-look at all those flecks of tissue in there. It looks kinda like dead brain. Smell it."

He jerked his head away from the observer scope. "You smell it, goddamn it. I'm not sticking my nose down there."

I scooped up some of the stuff with a retractor blade." Richard, I've been smoking cigars since I was 15- you know I can't smell a damn thing. Just sniff it.'

He took the retractor like it was booby-trapped, while I reached down to run some of the chalky fluid between my fingers. Gritty tissue in gritty liquid. It didn't have the slimy feel of all the pus I'd ever touched.

"If it's pus, it doesn't stink." He handed the retractor to Sally our scrub tech." Let's get the Path guys to do a smear of this stuff; they can at least tell us if it's infection."

There wasn't much to do while we waited; nothing to remove or repair and we damn sure weren't going to biopsy what was left of the spinal cord, so I just kept things wet with warm saline, watched the ugly fluid continue its slow ooze out of the cord, and tried to figure out how we were going to close this gaping hole. No way the swollen, distorted cord was going to fit back into the canal, so we'd need some type graft to help us close the dura in order to keep spinal fluid, liquified cord and blood from leaking out through the incision. I figured a piece of fascia from over the paraspinous muscles would be the best option; by the time we had a big strip harvested and Richard was suturing it down to the dural margins, Sally said, "Boss, pathology's here."

Dennis Burke, our favorite neuro-pathologist, had walked in quietly and was standing behind Richard, across the table from me. Dennis was the smartest guy in this or any other room and one of the nicest humans I'd ever met; also, a world class fly fisherman, rock climber, canoeist, you name it. He was also pretty much the cat's ass as a doc, a great guy who stood out among the pathologists who tended to be a strange group. When you looked objectively at Dennis, he was only about 5'5" tall but I never heard anyone mention it.

"Gentlemen, this is dead spinal cord. No infection, tumor, trauma, hemorrhage, no nothing. I'm going to guess it's some kind of weird spinal cord stroke; there probably aren't as many red cells as there should be in the pieces I got, but unless you want to whack out a bigger hunk for me to look at, that's where it sits."

I looked at Richard. Headshake, shoulder shrug, then we turned to Sally. "Suture, please, ma'am."

We hoped against all logic that just releasing the pressure from within her injured cord would make Maria better. It didn't. She awakened from the procedure unchanged and at the end of her first post-op week, remained completely paralyzed. The nurses taught her to communicate with eyelid blinks and she could shrug her shoulders weakly, but that was it. Seven days after the operation, Richard and I sat down with a translator and Maria's immediate family to explain the hopeless outlook. It was a miserable experience. The only dry eyes belonged to Delbert Riegel, the Jehovah's Witnesses Hospital Liaison. Riegel, a calm easy-going black man, was the formal interface between the Witness community and medicine. He spoke Spanish like a Mexican, English like a New Yorker and was sharper than your average car salesman. We'd spent a little time together during the hospitalizations of several members of his congregation, and while not exactly friends, we were usually on the same side. Both wanting the best for the patients, we just defined 'best" a little differently.

If Riegel wasn't up in the waiting area with Maria's family, I knew I could find him down in the cafeteria. He was a coffee nut and the only place on the premises that had anything he'd drink was downstairs. After the family conference, we sat in a corner booth while I apologized for the entire mess.

"I know this is terrible for everyone; I probably shouldn't have taken her to surgery without being positive she had a clot, but I thought it was the only real option. Now we're all up the proverbial creek with no paddle; we've got nothing else to offer and there's no way they're going to be willing to back off. Things aren't going to get any prettier- she's going to die, no matter what we do from here. Blood or no blood, that's all irrelevant now."

"Doc, the way the family sees the blood issue is pretty straight-forward, and no big deal. The ER missed that she was a Witness on the way in, but that's pretty understandable given the situation. I have a hunch you may have slipped in a transfusion or maybe two right before surgery – that would be after you knew she was a Witness, right? But I'll spot you those, because we all appreciate what you're trying to do, but that's it, OK? The bigger picture is that her people all know she's not going to make it, but that's not something we- or you- are going to do anything about, it just is what it is. No heroics, but we're all going to have to play this hand out. The other bad news is a different kind of worry. You know about her husband?"

"Only by rumor. He's supposedly a bad motor scooter who's in the pen for killing somebody, and from what Maria's mom says, he's not happy about things. It's pretty hard to blame him. He's got a 34-year-old wife who most likely is going to die a miserable death, just after giving birth to their third kid... and he's stuck in prison."

"The way the family talks that's about to change. He was convicted on a manslaughter charge and has been serving a four-year sentence. Maria got pregnant on one of their conjugal visits last year. He's got about 18 more months to serve but apparently, he's getting a compassionate early release -like tomorrow. Parole is a pretty short leash, but he'll be here in a day or so. I've never met the guy, but Maria's mom says he's a violent man. She's not happy about him being on the loose, especially with her daughter dying in front of his eyes."

"I guess she's not the only one."

Our Neurosurgery team rounded on its ICU patients twice daily; morning rounds at 0530 were "work rounds" for the residents and nurses. Afternoon rounds happened at anywhere from 4 to 6 whenever the day's surgery was done; they were for the entire team. This late walkaround was when we made plans, taught the younger residents, counselled families and shaped the service for the next 24 hours. The day after my talk with Riegel, I was late for the afternoon session, catching up with the team just as it boiled out of the ICU, headed for the family waiting room. I snagged Richard by his shoulder, pulling him out of the current of white coats. "What did I miss?"

'Not much. The brain tumor lady from this morning was a little slow to wake up but she's coming around. The broken back we're doing tomorrow is going to need a couple of units tonight. He says to tell you not to worry about the scar- he thinks his porn star days are over. Everybody else is pretty much status quo."

"What about Maria?"

"Hanging in there. She's got a little fever- about 38- probably from her urine because her lungs still look OK and both of the wounds are clean. Gary's bunch says everything is copacetic as far as the OB stuff goes. If this is going to go on much longer, I think we need to talk about a trach -if for no other reason just so she can kiss the baby."

"What her hematocrit like?"

"Down, as you would expect- about 24-25. I'll check it again in the morning."

"Don't. We're not going to give her any more blood, so no reason to drain any off. Did the husband show up?"

"Yup. He was in the unit right before we rounded. I didn't meet him, but the intern says he's a cold fish, a very cold fish. Two Texas Rangers brought him here."

'I can't wait."

Metropolitan Memorial had small conference-type rooms off the major waiting areas that were reserved for families of critically ill patients. Maria's family usually spilled over into two of these, but everybody crowded together when we came by to report after rounds. I picked out the new guy right away, primarily because the other family members left space around him even in the cramped room.; the pair of Rangers clinched the I.D. When we came in, he moved toward us while I elbowed my way to the front of our team so the two of us ended up face-to-face. Maria's mother, almost beside herself, introduced him in Spanish as Juan Carlos and then told him that I was the "chief doctor."

I offered my hand, but he ignored it, standing with hands in the pockets of his jeans. About 5' 8" and 150 pounds, he had black medium-length hair and a narrow face marred by acne scars and a tattoo of three tears below his left eye. His brown eyes were empty.

When Richard started his progress report Sanchez shifted his gaze momentarily, then resumed staring at me. Just to get everything out in the open I gave him a brief summary of everything that had happened, what we knew about Maria's disease and the dismal prognosis. He just maintained the hostile stare; later in the Army, I'd hear it called it "eye-fucking".

I wound things up by saying that because she was paralyzed, Maria needed help from the respirator to breath, which was why she had the tube down her throat. But going forward, I wanted to remove the tube and replace it with a tracheostomy, a tube we'd insert during a short surgical procedure through her skin and into her throat. This would make her breathing less labored, would allow her to mouth words and use her lips to take sips of water. It would also help the nurses to keep her lungs clean with suctioning. At the same time, we'd put a small tube through the wall of her abdomen into her stomach, so we could feed her. I finished up with, "We need to do both those things pretty quick, like tomorrow." His voice was low, soft and heavily accented. "When does she get well?"

"Unfortunately, she's not going to get well, Mr. Sanchez. The odds are almost 100% that she'll be paralyzed like this for the rest of her life. Her spinal cord was destroyed by what we think was a stroke." "What went wrong in the surgery?"

"The only thing that went wrong was that we didn't find the blood clot I'd expected. Her spinal cord was swollen and had been badly injured by the lack of blood flow, probably before she even came to the hospital. I was wrong about what was going on; we didn't make her any better with the operation, but we didn't make her any worse."

"I heard you gave her blood. She's a Witness- we don't take blood. It damns her to hell- do you know that?

"We didn't know she was a Witness when we transfused her. The pregnancy, the surgery to get your daughter out and the surgery on her neck would make her blood count dangerously low, so I believed she needed to be transfused. I've been over this with Maria's family and Mr. Riegel from your church. We didn't know she's a Witness; because she didn't consent to receive the blood, Mr. Riegel has told us - and your family - that the transfusion is not considered your wife's sin."

"That nigger doesn't know shit. I say it's a sin, just like cutting her up for no reason was a sin, and all of you will pay if she don't get well." His expression never changed.

Deep breath. "Mr. Sanchez, I'm sorry that's the way you feel. Everything we've done since Maria came to Parkland has been done to try to save her life and her baby's life. But you should know this: I've ordered everything that's been done. I made the doctors take the baby, I gave her the blood, I operated on her neck and I'm making the decisions about her care now. So, if you have a problem with the way we've cared for your wife, your problem is with me. And I'll be here every day."

"You're the boss, right? The big boss. Well, I do have a problem – a big problem. And I'll be here every day too. Big boss, you better hope she don't die." Then he walked away.

The next three days were a nightmare. Juan Carlos Sanchez wouldn't permit us to do anything to help Maria; no tracheostomy, no feeding tube, no nothing. He demanded to be in the room with her whenever she was examined, either by our troops or the OB guys; he terrorized the nurses on the night shift to the extent his escorts none-too-gently hustled him out and prevented him from visiting unless Richard or I okayed it. He refused to talk to anybody on the medical staff except me and raised hell if I wasn't on afternoon rounds.

The disruption was great enough that after talking with the hospital's administration I told Sanchez we were going to get a court order to bar him completely from the hospital if he didn't get with the program. He backed off a little then, but when one of the nurses reported that he'd been talking about how he'd killed a man who'd "crossed him," we had another sit-down with the Rangers and the hospital legal staff. They opined that we didn't have a case; so far, all he'd done was talk. Wonderful.

Meanwhile, Maria Elena Sanchez was slowly dying a pitiful death. Because of the endotracheal tube, we couldn't give her anything by mouth. She was getting ample fluids IV, but we couldn't keep up with her caloric needs through the nasogastric feeding tube. Neither of her surgical wounds were healing well but thus far she wasn't infected, although her skin was gradually beginning to break down at pressure points despite the nurses' heroic efforts to the contrary. And her gaunt, hollow face looked like a death mask.

Out of guilt and desperation I had every consultant in the house looking at her, the classical scenario of "futile care" before medicine had even given that charade a name. Juan Carlos Sanchez wouldn't talk to any of them, not that it mattered, but late in the week following her surgery, he did talk to me. After I'd finished the daily update, he said, "She's going to die soon."

"Yes, I think so. And if you won't let us do some of the things I've talked to you about, it won't be very long."

"You all have killed her; when she's gone I'm going to fix you." The Rangers hauled him out, and that was it.

During this terrible post-op period, no one ever heard him say a word to his wife. He'd touch her arm, caress her hair, wipe her tears, but he never spoke. He went to the Neonatal Care unit once to see his daughter. Juan Carlos scared the hell out of everyone.

Maria Elena Sanchez died during the night one day after my last talk with her husband. He was with her when her blood pressure dropped and she stopped triggering the ventilator. We didn't run a code, but there was a lot of excitement. By the time the ICU called me at home and I hustled in, Juan Carlos Sanchez had disappeared. He was just gone. The embarrassed Rangers didn't have a clue.

So, for a couple of weeks, everyone was pretty antsy, except I guess for me; I was scared shitless. A chief resident does a lot of coming and going at odds hours, and I must have seen Juan Carlos a hundred times; he was in the parking lot, on the road, at the gas station, everywhere. I started looking under my truck before I started it, even though I wouldn't have recognized a bomb unless it had a sign on it. After three days of jumping out of my skin, I decided I needed better protection.

At the time I had only one handgun, a huge Ruger Blackhawk in .357 magnum. This monster is an exact replica of the Old West six-gun and since Maria's death, I'd been lugging it around in my briefcase, but that wasn't going to do me much good if Sanchez decided to pay me a visit in the hospital. I took one of my old lab coats and cut a hole in the lining of the right pocket, so the six-inch barrel would fit down against my leg. Carrying the 2 1/2 pound pistol in my pocket made me look like either my shoulder was dislocated or I'd buttoned my coat all wrong, but at least for a couple of days I felt better about the whole thing.

That foolishness stopped one morning when the sheer weight of the damn gun caused it to rip through the coat's thin cotton lining and clang on the floor of the surgeons' locker room. It's a known fact -at least to gun nuts-that single action model Blackhawks like this one can't be made to discharge just by being dropped on an empty chamber, but I don't think the three guys in the locker room that day were convinced. On the other hand, they knew about the on-going Sanchez drama and after appropriate apologies they cut me a little slack. So, for a while afterwards I went back to toting the thing around in my briefcase. However, as weeks passed, and nothing happened I finally stuck the big pistol back under the bed and got on with being a brain surgeon.

Three months or so after Maria Sanchez' death I found a post-card in my hospital mailbox from Delbert Riegel. Juan Carlos Sanchez' escape had violated his parole with the Texas Department of Corrections, and subsequently he had been apprehended in Nogales Arizona as a part of a drug sting. There he'd been charged with "willful manslaughter ", whatever that means. It sounded to me that between Arizona and Texas he was going to be out of circulation for quite a while. I was leaving for the Army in a couple of months and thought Juan Carlos would probably have difficulty tracking me overseas, so I breathed a little easier.

Nonetheless, for 40 plus years, driving in or out of the hospital parking lot at night, my sub-conscious attention has been drawn to the occasional short slight guy hanging out at the adjacent bus stop or smoking near the staff entrance. I spend a little extra time just watching him before getting out of my truck, and from time to time, a minute or two thinking about the spring of 1975. Juan Carlos has long moved on to other issues, but I still remember the aura of menace that surrounded him, the fear that seeped into the ICU, and most of all,the sense of helplessness as we watched Maria Elena die.

CHAPTER SIX

Gun

I grew up in a little West Texas town. At the age of seven, I killed the first rattlesnake I'd ever seen with a BB gun. Hunting lizards along a dusty lane that led up to my dad's shop, I stumbled on this beast wiggling across bare dirt headed for the adjacent pasture. I was sure he was bigger than me but in real life he was maybe two and a half feet long, with a mean-looking triangular head and ten rattles. My air gun was an old style single shot; I had to load the BB and cock the spring before every shot, which usually took ten to fifteen seconds. On that day it took about five.

Snakes aren't very smart. If this particular viper had just bowed his neck and crawled in a straight line for the other side of the road, there would have been nothing I could have done to head him off. I damn sure wasn't going stand there while he crawled up to me, coiled and gave me the business, but every time I'd dance over in front of him, Brother Snake would reverse direction, giving me time and space for firing another shot. Hitting a reptile that size, even with an air gun, from ten paces is no great feat- assuming you can stop shaking long enough to aim- and within what seemed like an hour, but was probably about fifteen minutes, he had more than fifty copper spheres stuck in his skin. More importantly, now he was barely moving, and I was zeroed on his head. After another ten minutes or so he gave up the ghost, probably from either fatigue or copper poisoning.

After watching the motionless snake for another couple of minutes, I nudged him with the rifle's barrel then stomped on his head with my cowboy boot. That provoked a wiggle which provoked me to run empty my bladder before it went on automatic.

Back in action, I considered how to deal with the most important part of the post-mortem, that being the harvest of his rattles. In West Texas, you can't claim to have killed a rattler without having the proof; since my dad was out of town there was no chance I was walking away from that snake without his tail. Operationally, that was somewhat of a problem, since I was bereft of a knife. Three weeks earlier in the summer my knife-carrying privileges had been suspended after I made a mess of my left thumb trying to whittle the end of a mesquite branch into the head of a cane. I didn't know anybody that needed a cane, but the project had seemed reasonable at the moment.

So, absent a blade, I couldn't sever those rattles and the idea of biting them off with the tail wiggling was a non-starter. Only one thing left to my imagination, so standing on his head with the BB gun's muzzle firmly against the tail, I must have fired twenty rounds through the tough skin before the rattles fell loose. When I finally pocketed my trophy, that poor snake, from the tip of his crushed head through his copper -speckled body to the ragged stump of his tail, was barely recognizable. Still leery of touching him, I draped his body over my rifle's barrel and slung him across the fence into the pasture. This in honor of the long-standing myth that running over a dead rattler's head would cause a puncture of your tire and when you changed it, you'd die from just touching the poison. I didn't drive yet, but better safe than sorry.

When my dad came home the following day, I sprinted past my mother to his car, waving the gory rattlers and trying to tell the whole story before we got into the house. "You should have seen his fangs; when he hissed the poison dripped…" A little poetic license maybe, but still a pretty good tale, and I had the rattles. As the saying goes "It ain't bragging if you can back it up."

Dad listened thoughtfully. When I ran down, he said, "Boy, and with a BB gun. How many times did you have to shoot him?"

I was worried he was casting aspersions on my marksmanship, but we had a deal about telling the truth, so I answered, "Maybe a thousand, but I still had one packet of BBs left."

He looked at my mother and said, "I think your son is under-gunned." That Christmas, right before I turned eight, I got my first real rifle, a Winchester .22 single-shot. By the time I went back to school after the holidays, I'd shot five boxes of shells, two hundred and fifty rounds.

Firearms have been a significant part of my life ever since. Over the subsequent 65 years, I've hunted rabbits, squirrels, deer, racoons, feral hogs, quail, pheasant, dove, ducks, turtles, snakes and even a few more lizards. I've fired more rifles, shotguns and handguns than I can remember, plus one true machine gun (courtesy of the US Marine Corps). I've taken multiple weapons courses to include two self-defense series: "The Pistol in Self-Defense" and "The Civilian Shotgun", in addition to two Concealed Carry courses. I've had a valid Concealed Carry permit since the first year they were issued in Texas and was a card-carrying, dues-paying member of the National Rifle Association from 1977 to 2016.

Currently I belong to two gun ranges and shoot frequently at a Shooting Clays club. Many of my best memories are of teaching my two sons to shoot, hunting with them and finally being soundly trounced by them at the range with shotgun, rifle and pistol. I own three long gun safes, plus four handgun safes and for years have subscribed to my Marine son's motto that if you know how many guns you possess, you just don't have enough.

Not all my firearms experience has been theoretical. In 1975 as an Army doc assigned to Clark Air Force Base Hospital in the Philippines, I was forced to live off-base in a small community I'll call Lagunitas. The PI wasn't the Wild West it had been during the height of the Vietnam War, but despite marshal law, crime was rampant and violence endemic. Since the Air Force Base and the folks who worked there were the only real exception to poverty, Sutton's Law was prevalent; during the previous year the Base branch of the Bank of America had been robbed on payday.

Before I went over to the Philippines, the Air Force kindly paired me with an officer-advisor, a medical administrator who'd rotated back to the States six months earlier after completing a two-year tour at Clark. He provided a lot of important advice that was very helpful to a guy that couldn't find Manila on a map, but the last thing he told me in our two-hour talk was a potential life-saver. First, he asked me casually if I was a "shooter"; when I said, "Almost from birth," he then made certain I knew that for an active duty service member to possess an "undeclared" personal fire-arm was against Philippine, American and US Air Force regulations. The rumor was if you were found with such a firearm, your tour would be cancelled, and you'd be shipped back to your home base "in disgrace."

I was the only Army doc assigned to Clark; my regular duty station was ostensibly Tripler Army Medical Center in Honolulu, and I planned to exit the Army at the first possible opportunity anyway, so being sent home for having a personal handgun didn't sound like too much of a threat. When I told him so, my advisor replied, "If anybody asks, I never said this, but I wouldn't even think of living where you're going without a weapon. Just put the gun, along with a flashlight, in a spot where your house girl (the maid) can't find it but you can get to it at night. It can save your ass. Getting it in-country can be a bit of a hassle, but if you're shipping a POV (privately owned vehicle) over, there're lots of spots to conceal a handgun and a box of ammo. You'll end up selling the POV on the economy when your tour's up, but then just take the weapon down to the APs (Air Police) and tell them you'd forgotten about it. They'll give you some grief, but in the end, they'll ship it back with your household goods. Take the biggest thing you can comfortably shoot."

So, in early August 1975 I drove my Blazer cross-country to San Francisco for shipment overseas before I was scheduled to catch the Military Airlift Command flight out of Travis Air Force Base. On my way up the Peninsula, I sidetracked into the hills above Palo Alto to a trailhead I knew from college. With just a screwdriver and a wrench, I took the back off the driver's seat and made a spot for my Ruger .357 Magnum. Once the seat was back together I repeated the drill on the passenger's side, snuggling a box of fifty hollow-point rounds down into the backing then reassembling the seat. Finally, I coated each of the screwheads with a drop of clear fingernail polish, so on the other end I would know if someone had discovered my cache. Spy novel stuff.

Three weeks later, when I picked up the truck at the port of Manila, the polish was intact. After a quick stop in the parking area outside Clark's athletic fields, I stuffed the big pistol, now loaded, into the black doctor's bag that that Eli Lilly Co. gave every med student on graduation. Later I added a small mag light. The bag would sit on my bedside table for most of the next year, and just looking at it made me feel better about the whole situation.

About nine months into my thirteen months tour, my wife took some of her friends and the truck to Manila for a shopping week-end. I'd sold my motorcycle a month earlier, so, knowing I was going to need to catch a ride back from the hospital to our suburban outpost, I hauled the bag along when she dropped me off at the hospital that morning.

The transportation rules involving Clark and the surrounding Filipino community of Angeles City were a little bizarre, but necessary since experience had proven that nothing less than severe restriction of access to the base would prevent catastrophic pilferage of everything that wasn't nailed down. Consequently, once inside the Main Gate, you could get a "base taxi" that would carry you anywhere inside the wire. The taxis were abundant, clean, cheap and their drivers were fluent in English and very accommodating. But if you lived in a satellite community five miles out in the boonies, you were SOL. The base taxi could only go as far as the Main Gate and then you were, as the saying went, "on the economy."

The scene outside Clark's Main Gate in 1975 was a mirror image of the chaos that existed at that time on the Mexican side of every bridge crossing the Rio Grande River. Peddlers, food carts, money changers and a motley crew of street cleaners, beggars, hustlers, pimps and taxi drivers were a sure clue you weren't in Kansas any longer. Filipino taxis, in that era, were all garishly decorated Jeeps or Jeep knock- offs called jeepneys, featuring a driver's and a passenger's seat in front and a hopefully-padded bench seat in the rear. Lots of mirrors, beads and chains, maybe a lacy sun roof, but no doors, seat belts, luggage racks, fans, air conditioning, trip meter- nada. All trip prices were bargained in advance and sometimes subject to hostile re-negotiation en route.

Tips were expected to be paid before the passenger exited the vehicle, and any suggestions about navigation were severely discouraged. Just like Juarez in the 1950s.

Headed home on the day in question I picked the loudest driver with the lowest bid and we started walking to his jeepney. These were generally one-man operations, but on arrival somehow there were three of us; we'd been joined by a big, ugly tattooed dude with green teeth who my driver introduced as his "partner". Green Teeth vaulted into the back like he lived there, while the driver flicked his head in that direction and said, "No English." After he used a rag to brush off the passenger's seat, I climbed in and sat down. The driver looked over at the bag in my lap with a big grin. "You doctor, right?"

Not much to do but agree. He smiled at Green Teeth in the back and climbed behind the wheel. We hauled ass away from Main Gate on the regular route through the slums of Angeles City and pretty quick were on the single lane blacktop road that twisted almost aimlessly without apparent rhyme or reason through miles on miles of sugar cane.

Generally, jeepney drivers were anxious to chat their American passengers up, I guess to show off their command of English and hopefully increase the size of their tips, so the first sign I had that this might not be the routine commute was a cryptic back-and-forth between the two Filipinos in Tagalog. Just for my own clarification, I asked a couple of questions; the monosyllabic answers weren't wrong but seemed designed to cut any conversation short. By now I was really paying attention and popped the clasp on my bag. I didn't speak Tagalog, but I wasn't quite as ignorant as these fellas thought about the local road network.

Right after getting to Clark I'd bought a small motorcycle, a purchase that went against every safety principle supposedly engrained in a neurosurgeon's head. Bikes are unquestionably the most dangerous way to get from point A to point B; they are the only mode of modern travel in which the rider protects the vehicle. I could go on, but suffice it to say, they're not the routine transportation for your basic brain surgeon. However, it was cheap, looked like fun and I'd always had a little itch to ride, so what the hell. The first day I had the damn thing I was arrested at the main gate by the APs because I'd didn't have a license.

The problem was I'd never even been on a bike, and to ride on base you had to have a special license showing you'd passed a test administered by the base's mounted APs. These guys could really ride a motorcycle and the test they'd designed was a real bitch. A license wasn't required to ride off base (maybe one was, but I'd bet in the PI not one in a thousand riders were licensed) so after the embarrassing incident at the front gate, I taught myself to ride out on the roads that wandered through the sugar cane. By the time of my jeepney ride, the bike was history, but I knew almost as much about the local topography as my driver and his buddy. When we took a sharp right turn away from the route to Lagunitas on to a dirt track that ended in another barrio there weren't any more secrets.

I figured sooner was better than later, so I dragged the Ruger out. I didn't want the driver to underestimate my intensity, so I grabbed his shoulder with my left hand and showed him the big pistol, which by then was pointed right at his groin. No question that I had his attention right away, but suddenly the guy behind me, who I couldn't see at all, was scurrying around. Worried he might misread my intentions; I brought the gun up into his visual field and said, "Stop." When he ignored me, I very carefully pulled the .357s hammer back. The sound was really impressive, and now the muzzle was about six inches from the driver's right ear.

A cocked revolver is only five pounds of trigger pressure from exploding. On this road that was just one medium-sized pothole, and at least two of us understood that calculus immediately. The driver screamed something in Tagalog, then started jabbering in English at a rate I couldn't process. The jeepney came to a complete stop- a very careful one- at which point I could make out at least some of his conversation. "Please" was a lot of it.

By that time, I was shaking so badly I was afraid to try to de-cock the weapon, so I just dropped the driver's shirt and turned to point the big pistol at the guy in the back. He was busily trying to fold up his butterfly knife but looking up that muzzle made him stop everything but breathing. Him I really did want to shoot. Hell, I wanted to shoot them both.

The driver was still yammering away when I told his buddy to get out. Turns out the guy's English wasn't all that bad. With Green Teeth standing out in the weeds, we turned around and headed back for the turn to Lagunitas. It was a quiet, careful ride. By the time we got to the little barrio's gates, I had calmed down enough to safely de-cock the pistol, after which I carefully stuck it back in my bag, gave the driver the stink-eye and bailed out. He laid a little rubber, then yelled something over his shoulder that sounded a lot like "fuck you, round-eye". His heavy accent made it hard to be sure, but just on basic principles, I shot him the bird.

The laws of the Philippines and the tenuous legal standing of American service men stationed there being what they were, I told no one other than my wife the details of this encounter. Sure enough when my tour of duty was up, the APs reluctantly shipped my handgun back to the States without any hassle. The big pistol never left my bag for the remainder of my stay in the Philippines, but that single afternoon's experience crystallized a convincing argument in my head about the potential benefit of having a firearm and being willing to use it.

So, my life experience as a shooter, a hunter, a father, a teacher and a surgeon tells me that firearms can be used and enjoyed responsibly, that learning about guns, shooting and hunting can be a positive, maturing experience for young people, and that in the unlikely event that push comes to shove, the possession of a handgun and the will to use it can literally save your ass. But...

The societal cost of almost unlimited, uncontrolled access to firearms in this country is horrific. No segment of our society should be as aware of that fact as the medical profession; we're the final common pathway for all gunshot wounds and as such should be ashamed of our collective silence regarding the epidemic of gun violence in this country. The statistics are all old news, as are the shocking comparisons of other first-world countries' experiences with our own. What will never be old or stale or routine is the gruesome reality of a human brain destroyed by a lead slug.

To maintain that our society will ever successfully corral the psychological demons that drive mothers and fathers to shoot their children and children to kill their classmates is either an unrealistic pipe dream or a malicious lie. Similarly, we will never be able to identify and eliminate all the evils that motivate sniper wanna-bes, drug dealers and terrorist copycats. However, by facing a few simple facts we can make it one hell of a lot harder for each and every one of these deranged souls to destroy human life. Without trotting out the myriad of statistics that seem to accompany every discussion of the regulation of firearms, three such facts seem to be important.

Fact #1; Gun-related violence in America is a public health epidemic. It trails only motor vehicle accidents and drug overdoses as the greatest risk of death or disability to healthy Americans of every age. Like every epidemic, to control it we first must understand it in objective, clinical terms; to do that requires that gun violence be studied, without preconceived notions regarding its causes and potential cures. The mechanism to do that, in the fashion that we've successfully researched every other epidemic known to man, exists in the National Institutes of Health and its clinical arm, the Center for Communicable Diseases. Because of a law railroaded through Congress in 1996, federal funds are specifically prohibited for the study of this problem through these or any other research agencies, be they private or public. This is cynicism and / or stupidity of the most criminal degree.

Fact #2; Regardless of an individual's view of the constitutional framers' intent when the Second Amendment was drafted, no blanket right exists for individuals in this country to bear any and every type of firearm they may choose. That fact has been reaffirmed on multiple occasions by the formal prohibition of a variety of weapons for individual purchase or possession. Subsequently, those prohibitions have withstood every legal challenge based on constitutional grounds. Implicit in these successes is the society's right to protect itself from the indiscriminate use of weapons whose capacities for destruction have proven to be beyond the imagination of even the most futuristic thinker of the 18th century.

Fact 3#: The individual rights enumerated in the Bill of Rights are routinely subject to regulation by Federal and state governments when the health and well-being of society members is clearly at risk. That's why we license individuals to drive a car, fly a helicopter, practice medicine or cut your hair. The belief that no such guarantee of a minimal level of competence and safety should be necessary for the purchase and use of a firearm is ludicrous. That is the very purpose of government.

Somewhere beyond what's legal and what's legacy, our society has to search for what's right, what best serves the needs and the safety of its members while conforming to the baselines of our democracy that were established two and a half centuries ago. If we're willing to study the problem of firearm-related violence objectively, then craft appropriate regulations that focus on the causative issues discovered, to potentially include firearms capabilities, consumer access, mandatory education and appropriate licensing among others, we will have made an important step in addressing this public health hazard.

I realize there are over 300,000,000 privately-owned firearms in America, but this number is deceiving, and doesn't mean 300 million owners. A large percentage of these weapons is clustered in the hands of confessed "gun nuts" like me, individuals who are willing to be held accountable for their firearms' safety and security and for their own competence. When all the political rhetoric is dispelled, these are your basic solid citizens who recognize the validity of both sides of this debate and strongly believe there's not an "either or" solution.

For everybody else, I'd recommend a mandatory evening or two with GSW victims and their families in a big city ICU.

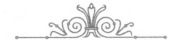

CHAPTER SEVEN

VA

I first went to the regional Veterans' Administration Hospital as a wet-behind-the -ears neurosurgery resident in 1972, just as our medical school assumed responsibility for medical staffing of the hospital. The pre-existing medical staff- all fulltime VA employees- stayed on, usually until retirement; consequently, the presence of essentially two parallel medical staffs made for some interesting interactions.

Dr. Kerrell Cooper was, at that time, the sole full-time Dallas VA neurosurgeon, having been in his job since leaving active duty at the end of the Korean Conflict in 1953. Dr. Cooper had trained at the Mayo Clinic during and immediately after WW ll, then been assigned to a sequence of military hospitals to serve out his four-year obligation. Unfortunately, just as he was about to "get out", Korea flared up and he was retained for the duration of that conflict. Apparently the job market for neurosurgeons in 1953 was soft and he ended up at the new VA facility in Dallas, practicing by himself. So he stayed, and stayed.

When I knew him twenty years later, Dr. C was in a chronic state of being pissed off, perhaps due to being involuntarily extended by the Army way back when, or maybe, because, after being stuck in the VA system for two decades, it suddenly was treating him like sour milk. For whatever reason, he wasn't very interested in cooperating with the new boys on the ward, me and my chief resident Harvey Birsner, a wild man who'd just gotten out of the Navy himself.

In fairness, Dr. Cooper wasn't really interested in practicing neurosurgery any longer, as long as he came away with a paycheck every two weeks. He showed up to work late, left early and went on vacation ("leave") whenever the hell he wanted. For a while, there at the beginning, we'd politely ask if he'd like to make rounds with us or come to the clinic to see a few patients or even come to the OR, but it wasn't happening, and most of the time he didn't bother with an excuse. Just "No." So we just stayed out of each other's way, more or less.

Harvey, who became a close friend during our six months together, basically wrote Dr. Cooper off as the "laziest man I've ever met". He wanted nothing to do with the older guy's opinions or advice and made no attempt to hide those feelings. On the other hand, things were different from my worms-eye point of view. I was 18 months out of my internship, could still barely spell "neurosurgery" and almost every day was seeing some new disease or running into a new patient management problem, whereas Dr. C had been practicing neurosurgery since I was five years old. Like it or not, he'd seen it all and every modification a million times over, so I had no problem asking for his input, even though frequently he made it clear I was a real dumbass-which was not far from the actual state of affairs.

As a result, the two of us developed a tenuous teacher- pupil relationship, one which I took great care to cultivate because, not only did the guy know more than I was going to learn in the next four years, but also when my chief resident was out of town looking at jobs or off chasing a sequence of pretty recovery room nurses, I frequently was sorely in need of back-up ...and both Dr. C and I knew it.

Like a lot of professionals of his age, Dr. Cooper smoked like a steam engine. The VA hospitals were notorious for permitting and even encouraging smoking. In the 1970s cigarettes were 35 cent a pack in the hospital's PX, and smoking was permitted on the wards, in the waiting rooms, in the ER and in all the physician's lounges. It was not uncommon to see a group of doctors making rounds with lit cigarettes, so usually when I took Dr. C to see a patient, I'd have to ask him to put out his smoke before going in the patient's room. As bizarre as this seems today, it was simply a sign of the times, but with Dr. Cooper it had an interesting surgical application.

One of the more common brain tumors in older adults is a very bad actor known as a glioblastoma, a malignant tumor that even today is incurable. The treatment plan for these lesions is first to remove as much as is possible surgically and then to follow-up with radiation therapy, but even with the addition of sophisticated chemotherapy regimens, the mean life span after diagnosis is still less than two years. These tumors are malignant growths of the support cells of the brain itself; as such, they are in and a part of the brain tissue. In addition, they are very vascular. Consequently, there is no way to surgically "get around" one of the tumors without taking out enormous amounts of normal brain tissue, which is complicated by the fact they usually bleed like stink. So, surgery of glioblastomas in 1972 usually amounted to either just a cautious little biopsy or a real blood bath- no real middle ground.

We had a patient with one of these tumors on the surgery schedule on a day when my partner Harvey called in sick. Bright and early, I was in the OR, telling the scheduling nurse we were going to have to cancel for lack of adult supervision, when Dr. Cooper, having his second cup of coffee and third cigarette of the morning, heard me talking and interjected that he'd be happy to scrub in on this one to "show me the ropes". Other than me, the poor patient had no idea who was doing his surgery, so there was no mechanism, graceful or not, to refuse this offer.

While the OR sent for the patient, I collected all his x-rays and displayed them on a view-box for my new attending surgeon. The most important piece of evidence was the arteriogram I'd done the day previously, a study that revealed a myriad of abnormal vessels diagnostic of this tumor type. Dr. C grunted; when I asked what he thought, he said," Yup, it's a GBM; looks like a two smoker to me."

He waited to pounce on my next question, but I just said," Yes sir" and went to scrub. It's hard to get in too much trouble with your mouth closed.

Operatively, things went about as expected. Dr. C was decent help as, without any forced errors, I exposed the brain surface where the tumor was located, then with great trepidation removed a tiny sliver of what appeared to be abnormal brain to send to Pathology for a frozen section. Stopping the resultant bleeding was a major undertaking, but after charring the surrounding cortex with the cautery for ten minutes I was making some progress when the pathologist came back in to confirm our diagnosis. Glioblastoma.

Dr. C looked at me over his bifocals. " Now what, junior?"

I confessed I thought we should probably just close up and go home, because 1) we had a diagnosis, 2) we weren't going to cure this patient, and 3) I was sure he'd bleed to death if we did anymore.

"Naah- all you've done is piss it off. Now, it'll swell up like a poisoned pup. We need to get a bunch of this thing out. Just open up that cortex right across there, junior, then suck like hell."

Well, under Dr. Cooper's constant nagging, I ultimately made a huge cavity in that gentleman's brain. After I had sucked out at least a fistful of tumor, the arteries down in the hole were literally pumping blood. The blood pressure started down, anesthesia was transfusing, and I was sweating bullets, chasing down and coagulating the biggest bleeders. Finally, with most of the major arteries under control, the geyser-like action subsided but the entire surface of the cavity continued to weep blood faster than my suction would remove it. My very small bag of tricks was empty, so I looked over at my assistant. He just shook his head in disgust and said, "Gotta pack it," reaching up to the Mayo stand for a monstrous handful of surgical gauze, which he moistened then stuffed into my excavation. That wasn't enough, so he forced a second handful down on the first, irrigated the packing, then stripped off his gloves. Telling the scrub nurse to get me some warm irrigation-" Real warm, honey"- he went out the door fumbling for his cigarettes. The last thing I heard was, "Stay with it, now-junior".

Seventeen minutes later by the clock- two smokes' time- Dr. C scrubbed back in. We'd dropped a couple more units of blood, but the pressure had come back up, and the patient's heart rate had settled back to normal. I cautiously took the laundry out, one wad at a time, then coagulated a few small bleeders, but there was nothing left to do. We had a diagnosis, we'd removed a large amount of tumor and all the hemorrhage was controlled; time to go home. In the recovery room, the patient wasn't much worse for having his brain treated like his liver, and by the next day he was back to his pre-op status. Dr. Cooper actually made rounds that day, looked the guy over, then nodded his head. "A two smoker, like I said."

I never developed a taste for cigarettes but seventeen minutes by the clock can be pretty sound theraputic advice when the chips are down. Admittedly, this is not a technique I've used routinely in my surgical practice, but it has saved at least four lives when nothing else would work. Gauze packing under pressure has proven especially effective in dealing with large penetrating wounds of the brain secondary to gunshot wounds or shrapnel. In fact, my next survivor was a young Special Forces sergeant wounded in Thailand in late 1975. Three days post-op, while we were waiting to finally load him on the bird for Hawaii, I told the Green Beret that Dr. C would say he was a "two smoker." He looked at me for a moment, then said, "Doc, don't take this wrong, but you surgical dudes are weird." And he didn't even know Dr. Cooper.

Despite my appreciation for the old neurosurgeon's advice, it's a fact of life that over the last fifty years, the VA has become the refuge of some of the laziest health care professionals in captivity. Nurses, aides, schedulers, administrators, x-ray technicians, and yes, doctors like my old mentor- a large cadre of slackers dedicated to doing the least amount of work over the shortest period of time for the maximum amount of money. These are people who really, despite their protestations to the contrary, don't give a rat's ass about the veteran patients that make up the VA's population, or the other providers on the health care team. They're the reason a VA operating room can only do one-third the number of cases a university hospital OR can do in a day; the reason that VA out-patient clinics can only see 40% of the patient load normally processed through a private practice clinic in the same time frame. These slugs have taken a system intended to provide good medical care for folks who deserve it and have been a large factor in perverting it into a huge, inefficient bureaucratic mess whose primary mission is self- preservation. Thank god they're still in the minority.

On Sunday 6 April 1975, I was completing medical charts in the small doctor's office on the Neurosurgery floor at the Dallas Veterans' Medical Center. It was late, I was tired and having second thoughts about giving my junior resident the day off, even if he hadn't seen his wife and new baby much during the last busy week. I hated doing those damn charts.

When Wesley, the floor's head nurse, peaked in the door then came in and sat down, I was elated to have some human company, his especially. Wes was an old timer; he'd been an VA fixture long before I showed up in 1972. He knew everything and everybody worth knowing at the 600-bed hospital. Routinely keeping us out of trouble with the suits on the first floor, he maintained a high level of nursing care and enthusiasm in an environment renown for personnel shortages and slipshod work ethics. Wes was a gem, probably in his early 60s with a forever wife, two daughters he'd put through law school and a generous guaranteed pension. If Wesley wanted to talk, I wanted to listen.

I asked him how his weekend was going; with tears in his eyes, Wes he said it was the two worst days of his life. This man never whined, and he wasn't whining now, but he could barely speak. His younger daughter, who worked for the Defense Department, had been sent to Saigon as a caregiver to one of the orphans on the first flight of Operation Baby Lift, the planned evacuation of over a thousand Vietnamese orphans in the face of the impending fall of Saigon. The US Air Force C5-A had taken off from Tan Son Nhut airfield on Friday afternoon, but developed engine trouble en route to Clark Air Force Base in the P.I. After attempting to return to Tan Son Nhut, the big plane had crashed on a repeat approach. Out of 328 souls on board, there were 124 deaths; Wesley's daughter had been one of them. She was 27 years old. He just sat there looking at me.

Wesley was in the hospital for the 4-12 shift a day after his daughter's death because he hadn't been able to find a stand-in among the ward's usual nursing cadre and wasn't willing to turn the shift over to a nurse that didn't know his patients. There was nothing I could say, other than how sorry I was. It sounds as hollow now as it did that night. We talked briefly- I can't even remember about what- then he got up, said I should "get on home to the family," and went back to work. Forty-three years later, I still struggle to understand this almost inhuman act of selflessness.

What I do understand is that some of the most dedicated nurses I've met over my practice life have been career VA employees. These selfless stars could have worked anywhere and been recognized as the cream of the crop in any hospital system in this country, but they chose to stay at the VA; less money, worse working conditions, a stultifying professional environment and less than zero administrative support. They'll tell you they stayed because 1) they were desperately needed and 2) because of the patients. There has never been enough of this type nurse and there are fewer every year.

There's been another change in the VA over the past twenty years that few are willing to discuss, and that's the change in the VA's patient population. The vets I took care of who served both before, during and immediately after Vietnam seemed to share a common cultural milieu. Regardless if they came from rural areas, small towns or the big city, they were generally employed, most with families but just not sufficient money to pay for health care insurance. Routinely, they pitched in to help on the wards where we were always short-handed. They were polite to and appreciative of the hospital's nurses, LVNs and orderlies and far more understanding than the medical staff of the "make-do" philosophy imposed on the VA system by Washington D.C.'s shifting priorities. "Just like the Government," they'd say, shaking their heads, when we ran out of toilet paper, clean linens or eggs for breakfast. Generally, above all else, these guys wanted just to get out of the hospital, go home and get back to work. Interestingly, almost all these veterans had been drafted into service.

That dynamic began to change sometime in the late 1980s; most marked was the sudden appearance of a not-too-subtle sense of hostility between the veteran patients and the entire hospital system. Part of that was wholesome; chronic objections to appointment delays, long clinic and surgical wait times, difficulties with pharmacy services, and restrictions on rehabilitation services all became much more strident and open. When the lethargic VA bureaucracy failed to respond, as it had forever, a tsunami of complaints went to veterans' organizations, Congress and to the media. The VA administrative cockroaches started scuttling for cover, and problems that had existed for decades began to become instant scandals. Unfortunately, despite the subsequent thrash, it's not clear that all the noise has made significant differences in important parameters of care.

Another, less healthy aspect of change involved not the veterans' conflict with the system but the patients' conflict with their caregivers. Like it or not, medicine boils down to one human being's attempts to heal another's sickness, mitigate his/her pain and manage his / her disability; as flawed as we all are, that's a two-part contract. For whatever reason, in the recent past, many veterans have begun to welch on their part of that deal. They've become less dependable in honoring their appointments, less truthful regarding their signs and symptoms, less cooperative in following medical instructions and less reliable in their own health maintenance. Simultaneously, many have come to treat the VA caregivers as opponents, as "parts of the problem" as opposed to potential allies in finding solutions. These traits set up an adversarial system that all too often results in dissatisfaction on both sides of the equation.

It's ironic that while many politicians seem to believe the remedy for the nation's health care problems is a nationalized health system patterned on the VA, a different set of politicians, veterans and so-called health care experts seem to feel the solution to the VA's undeniable problems lays in enabling veterans to seek their health care outside of the VA system on the private health care market at the government's expense. There are multiple issues with both these approaches, many of which are beyond the limited scope of my expertise, but from a guy that's worked in both systems, here are a few that come quickly to mind.

1) Cost: The estimated cost of adding a significant number of veterans to the private patient population would be enormous if the patients were charged the going private insurance rates. If however, they were charged the current VA costs or simply Medi-Care rates, many private physicians would refuse to admit them to their practices, just as an increasing number of physicians refuse to accept Medi-Care, because of the low reimbursement rates and the sheer hassle (and expense) of dealing with the government system.

2) Physician Choice: This doesn't exist in the VA system, so theoretically the ability to choose one's own provider would be a definite improvement. Looked at in detail, maybe not so much.

What physicians actually will want to accept VA patients (see #1) and assuming willingness, who should be eligible to treat these patients? (see #3).

3) Quality Control: The changes that have come about in the VA system since 1970 have significantly upgraded the required qualifications of physicians practicing in that system. Some, perhaps even many, may be lazy but at least on paper they are qualified. The same cannot be said for the stew that is the private practice of medicine in the USA. Taking into consideration that any VA payment system would almost certainly provide low-end physician reimbursement levels, the physicians most likely to be attracted to this new patient population would be those less competitive, generally meaning less competent, in the open market.

4) Medical Malpractice: In essence, physicians employed by the VA system are indemnified against medical malpractice litigation. A patient can file a claim alleging malpractice against a VA doctor, but the suit itself is against the Veterans Administration; any financial awards are the responsibility of the VA itself. With annual malpractice premiums for neurosurgeons above $300,000 in many locations, there are obvious legal disincentives for physicians to accept greater potential liability for reduced compensation.

5) Continuity of Care: For all its admitted shortcomings, the VA provides a truly integrated system of health care. The VA patient from Dallas who needs medical care in Sheridan Wyoming or moves to Orlando FL has his /her entire medical record, to include imaging studies and medication history, available to the new health care providers just by opening his/ her computerized medical record. There's no question of system compatibility or user stupidity; it's all right there, chapter and verse, totally independent of the patient's memory or the prior institution's cooperation. This system currently needs an upgrade, but it's the best around.

Like so much of America's health care system the Veterans Administration is a mixed bag. I don't believe it's the right model for a makeover of our national health care program nor do I think it is the fetid morass it's currently portrayed to be. If the VA is to be improved, the effort will require input,energy, and "buy-in" from all of the players, to include the newer generation of patients. At a minimum, the system needs and deserves more hard-nosed oversight as well as thoughtful, focused re-structuring with the duals goals of providing a consistently higher quality of care as well as more bang for the taxpayer's buck. What the VA hospital system doesn't deserve is mindless destruction at the hands of a lynch mob of poorly-informed, self-interested, publicity-hungry zealots, a mob which unfortunately includes a vocal minority of patients, physicians and politicians.

CHAPTER EIGHT

Witness

Throughout my neurosurgical practice I've had repetitive encounters with Jehovah's Witnesses as patients, and contrary to organized medicine's party line, these experiences have been almost uniformly positive. While I don't share the Witnesses' weird philosophical / religious convictions, (which seem to me to be based on perverted interpretations of obscure isolated Old Testament scripture), I respect the strength of their community and the support it offers to its membership in its ongoing struggle with the mores of modern medicine.

For operational clarity, let's just say that Witnesses believe that to willingly accept human blood or blood products in transfusion is a mortal sin. That relatively simple stance can be and is parsed in a plethora of ways, so if you've got a Witness patient- especially one you plan to operate- it's important to know exactly what flavor of Witness is on the schedule. Are some blood products OK and if so what are they? How about cell-free serum or plasma concentrate? Are just red blood cells forbidden? What constitutes "transfusion", meaning can you bank the patient's own blood and give it back at a later date? Can you scavenge blood at the OR table with what's called a Cell Saver and then re-infuse the spun red cells? Gotta know the rules if you're gonna play the game.

Generally, when a surgeon is dealing with a Witness patient, he / she will also be dealing with an appointed representative of the

Witness community (known as the hospital representative) who will have some degree of medical sophistication and consequently will be able to articulate the patient's, and the patient's family's, medical wishes. However, it's critically important for the surgeon to verify what the hospital rep has said when alone with the patient, since if push comes to shove, it's going to be just the doc and the patient, who may actually care more about living than hewing to the party line.

All of the above relates to elective surgery or at least to situations in which a surgeon can actually consult with a patient prior to being involved in his / her care. Unfortunately, neurosurgeons often become treating physicians in emergency situations in which the patient is unable to communicate at all, and not infrequently there is no family available and no evidence of a prior medical directive.

All practicing Witnesses are supposed to carry such a directive on their persons -the so-called "blood card"- a signed document stating that even at peril of the signee's life, he/ she refuses blood and blood product transfusion. As a rule, legal authorities have recognized these cards as valid health care directives and currently most ERs instruct their medical personnel to routinely search patients' possessions for them, but if you've ever been in a busy ER you'll understand why it's still a rare occurrence when Witnesses are identified by this documentation alone prior to medical intervention. It's also pretty clear, from the official church's point of view, that transfusing an unconscious Witness in an emergency situation doesn't confer any ethical guilt on the patient. Said differently, assuming that decision has been made without the patient's consent, no negative karma is incurred. The same cannot be said for the legal jeopardy that physicians in this situation may experience. Currently, there has been no consistency in court rulings in the few cases litigated to date, which translates as a real potential risk for docs that knowingly elect to breech patients' explicit desires regarding transfusions.

Where the rubber meets the road here is in the management of children, so naturally my first encounter with the Witness community came in the person of a five year old boy I'll call Raoul. This was during the final year of my residency when I had the responsibility of managing indigent kids with neurosurgical problems at our Children's Hospital.

Raoul, a cute Latino kid, had dropped out of pre-school about a month before I saw him because of increasing headaches, nausea and recent vomiting. The clinic's chief pediatrician, a senior resident just like me, had smelled a rat and even though Raoul was tough to examine, he felt that he could identify evidence of an abnormally high intra-cranial pressure. This is done by a careful evaluation of the patient's fundi and is no slam dunk, even in a cooperative adult, but this pediatrician was a whiz. After multiple attempts he decided Raoul had it.

The skull is a closed bony box with only one real opening through which passes the spinal cord and two important arteries. Other almost minuscule openings allow the nerves that control smell, vision, hearing and the muscles and sensation of the face to transit. The bony box is filled to the brim with brain, spinal fluid and blood in the arteries and veins of the brain. If anything extra, like a tumor, is added to the contents of the box, the pressure within goes up. In a short while, that increase is reflected in the optic nerve head located beneath the retina. The increased pressure also distends the brain's covering - known as the dura mater, which is exquisitely sensitive and begins to complain. Ergo, headaches.

My suspicious pediatrician got a technicism brain scan of Raoul, because that was state of the art in 1975, a scan which proved we had a real problem. Not only was there a tumor about the size of a large walnut, but it was located right smack in the middle of the main passageway for spinal fluid, meaning both the mass of the tumor itself and the consequent blockage of spinal fluid flow was elevating Raoul's intra-cranial pressure. A double whammy for this nice kid.

The only good news was that Raoul's age, plus the location and appearance of the tumor, made us almost certain this was a benign type of tumor known as a ependymoma which has its origin from the cells lining the brain's spinal fluid chambers. If the tumor could be completely removed surgically without injury to any critical brain anatomy, Raoul could be cured. Two important caveats: 1) The approach to the tumor was pretty tricky, and 2) ependymomas bleed like stink.

At this point in my training (about three months before completion) I'd done about 100 intra-cranial cases, mostly tumors and blood vessel problems, with relatively good results and a small number of real disasters. Most of this good fortune was due directly to the seven months I'd spent in Zurich Switzerland with Professor M.G. Yasargil, a Turkish-born, Swiss-trained neurosurgeon who was completely re-writing the book on operative neurosurgery. Although several other surgeons had dabbled with applying the operating microscope to brain surgery, Yasargil made it the center piece of his operative technique and in a shockingly short time developed a technical mastery the world had never even imagined. My opportunity to be in the OR watching this genius as he made one quantum leap after another in treating previously fatal diseases was the seminal point in my career, an experience that irrevocably changed my life.

I had assisted the Professor as he removed two ependymomas (one in a small child) and as I did after every operation, I'd written copious notes about every step in the process, so while I didn't have any delusions about being Yasargil, I did know the drill and, as I mentioned, it wasn't my first rodeo.

So, talking to Raoul and his folks, I was confident I could take his tumor out, relatively sure I could do it without hurting him, but not at all sure I could do it without losing enough blood to make a transfusion absolutely necessary. I explained all of the above to Raoul's parents and to Delbert Riegel, the Witness Hospital Rep. I said I wouldn't transfuse Raoul unless I had to, but if that happened I wanted their permission to give him blood. They flatly refused.

Raoul's mother and father not only refused permission for transfusion, they refused permission for the operation. I could see the decision was killing them, but they said it would be preferable that he not have the surgery and die than to commit the mortal sin of allowing him to be transfused. They wanted to take him home. I didn't even have kids then, and I couldn't believe it.

As you know, there's a legal way to deal with this issue. The doc, or the hospital, calls Child Protective Services, explains the situation and CPS calls an on-call judge who promptly transfers custody of the kid to CPS, whose representatives sign the op permit. The Witnesses then get an opposing ruling to restore the child to the parents' custody, by which time the operation is over and ideally everything is copacetic. At this point, Raoul's hematocrit was 40%, on the lower end of normal for his age, but damn sure good enough to go through a relatively bloodless operation. The problem was that this procedure promised to be anything but bloodless, especially in the hands of a guy doing his first one, so despite the good relationship I thought I'd developed with the parents I really didn't have any choice. Together with the pediatric chief resident I went through the steps to get CPS involved.

All well and good... except Raoul didn't cooperate. The night prior to the scheduled operation he spiked a temp to 102; despite a rushed fever work-up we couldn't find a source. I cancelled the procedure and the following day our custody order was reversed. Raoul went back to the custody of his parents who proceeded to check him out of the hospital Against Medical Advice, or almost check him out, because with the help of Delbert I convinced them to let him stay until we found and treated the source of his fever.

That took a couple of days – he had a UTI- and by the time the pediatricians got on top of his infection he taken a definite turn for the worse as regards his brain tumor. Now he was listless, complained of continual headache and had such nausea and vomiting that he was becoming dehydrated. The peds guy stuck an IV in him, but we still couldn't get over the transfusion hump with his parents. He was dying right in front of their eyes; they were miserable, I was miserable, and the pediatrician was miserable.

In a break from discussing this with the parents, Delbert told me that if I'd promise not to transfuse their son unless I knew he was going to die right there on the OR table, he thought the parents would give me permission to operate. In the meanwhile, my peds buddy had gone back to the judge through CPS, but she'd been unhappy with the whole song and dance. Apparently, he'd let some harsh words slip over the telephone, after which she'd gotten pissy and "provisionally" turned down CPS' request "awaiting more information."

Delbert convinced me to take another shot, so I made the promise and the parents consented very reluctantly over the protests of other members of the congregation, none of whom had a damn bit of skin in the game. By this time Raoul's hematocrit was in the high thirties and the plan was looking sketchier by the minute.

Regardless of any promises to the contrary, I had the kid typed and crossed for four units, two of which were in the OR when we put him to sleep. The moment things got just a little wet I was going to give him more blood than I could lose, and worry about the parents, the judge and the pediatrician further down the road.

Long story short, the surgery went like a dream. We lost zero blood on opening, the tumor almost extruded itself when I got the ventricle open and all its blood supply was located in one small pedicle that I isolated, coagulated and cut. The damn thing just about dropped out on my lap. We got in and out in about three hours, which was smoking fast for me, and Raoul woke right up in Recovery where his first post-op hematocrit was 33%. Halleluiah.

We were all still celebrating on Raoul's second post-op day when he developed belly pain, vomited bright red blood and began to pass black diarrheal stools. Over about six hours his crit dropped to 25% and it became obvious he'd developed a stress ulcer, probably at the junction of his stomach and duodenum.

The general surgeons weren't amused by our little morality play. They wouldn't touch him until he'd had two units of fresh blood and there were four more in the OR refrigerator. The parents refused to talk to me, and when I got that self-same judge on the telephone, she tore a large bloody chunk out of my butt. Nonetheless we got Raoul to the OR that night and according to the general surgeon, it was "a piece of cake."

Raoul's folks took him home a week later. During that time they'd regained custody and refused to let me see the kid. His post-discharge neurosurgical care came through the office of a sympathetic private guy in town; I never saw the boy again. Four years later when I'd come back from the Army, the private neurosurgeon called just to let me know that Raoul was doing well, although he'd developed hydrocephalus after my operation and had needed a shunt. Now almost four years later his CT scan showed no evidence of recurrent tumor.

When I returned from the service Delbert Riegel morphed into a one-man PR firm, so I started getting a reasonable number of consultation requests from Witnesses around the Southwest. Ove the next decade I'd accumulated about twenty Witness patients for intra-cranial surgery, all but one of whom had had good outcomes. The patient who did poorly was a lady in her late 40's who suffered a ruptured intra-cranial aneurysm and was pretty sick when she was transferred to us some six days later. She badly needed an operation to obliterate the aneurysm and prevent a second almost surely fatal hemorrhage, but her family refused permission to transfuse and the outside surgeon refused to do the operation without blood.

The aneurysm itself wasn't an overwhelming problem; knowing the guy who sent her, I figured he was a bigger potential threat than the aneurysm itself. But by the time we got Angela in transfer, her hematocrit had drifted down to the low 20s. Any other patient I would have transfused a couple of units before we went to the OR, but that wasn't going to happen, so we tuned her up with some plasma expanders and then were ultra-cautious with her procedure.

On her first post-op day her crit dropped to 19% then appeared to stabilize so I figured we were probably out of the woods. No such luck.

The blood that escapes during an aneurysmal hemorrhage gets packed tightly along the small arteries at the base of the brain, and as it begins to breakdown, the chemicals released produce an intense narrowing of the adjacent arteries, a narrowing severe enough to markedly reduce blood flow through these vessels. This process, known as "vasospasm", usually begins around day 7 post-hemorrhage and with the exception of re-hemorrhage is the major cause of mortality in these patients, That timetable makes getting the aneurysm dealt with early after the initial hemorrhage very important, because the most effective treatment for vasospasm, until recently, has been the artificial elevation of the patient's blood pressure to very high levels, a procedure which increases blood flow through the spastic arteries and often, but not always, can prevent severe brain injury, death or permanent disability. Ironically when we artificially raise the pressure, we like the hematocrit to be in the low 30s, because that facilitates blood flow through small vessels, but we definitely don't like it down in the teens, which is where Angela's hematocrit was settling out.

Because we could see the thick layer of blood around her arteries both by CT and through the scope at surgery, it was a cinch she was going into spasm. I warned her family after the operation that if they had any second thoughts about changing our rules of engagement this was the time to let me know. They were adamant they wanted to stay the course, and I honored their wishes. Angela developed multiple strokes, followed by severe brain swelling and died four days post-op.

I don't know for a fact that giving Angela three units of blood and keeping her hematocrit around 30 would have made a difference but it would have been the right thing to do medically. I guess I'm convinced it wouldn't have been the right thing for Angela, but the fact I'm still turning it over in my head twenty years later suggests my conviction is less than solid.

Maria is the last Witness patient I'll tell you about and perhaps the most perplexing. She'd come to medical attention because at the age of 56 she'd developed epilepsy. When the appropriate tests were done it was found that she had a large blood vessel-type tumor located in her left temporal lobe. This abnormality is called a cavernous angioma and is sort of a like a birthmark in the brain tissue. It is fragile and bleeds easily, but unlike aneurysms and arterio-venous malformations, the bleeding is venous, meaning under very low pressure and usually easily stopped simply by the pressure of the surrounding brain matter. However, the ultimate breakdown of the hemoglobin molecules in the free blood produces an iron molecule which is very prone to cause seizures. Given that the temporal lobe itself is perhaps the most seizure prone region of the brain, it wasn't a big surprise that Maria had developed "fits". The treatment of choice for both the cavernoma and the "fits" was to remove the abnormality along with the ring of blood-stained brain around it.

These things don't bleed much when you're taking them out, so as long as the surgeon can get to the cavernoma without damaging any brain and is careful in the removal process, the operation is safe and effective, meaning there will be no more hemorrhaging and 75-80% of patients will be seizure free off medications.

I went through the routine pre-op stuff with Maria and her husband, both of whom were adamant that she receive no blood or blood products. The Witnesses had come up with a new written "disclaimer" which she requested be part of her chart. It stated that even if her life was judged by me to be in danger, she stated unambiguously that she refused transfusion of any type.

By this time in my career, I was pretty comfortable about assessing operative risk and even more comfortable with mentally-competent adults making their own health care decisions; I also figured on my worst day there was no way I could screw up Maria's surgery badly enough that she'd die without a transfusion, so away we went. Her chart was clearly marked "NO BLOOD PRODUCTS" and before the anesthetic started I made sure everyone in the room knew we were going bloodless on this one. Maria's operation wasn't exactly a walk in the park, but I wasn't in a cold sweat when I got the malformation out, and as my trusty resident began to close, I figured we'd lost maybe 100 cc. total. She'd started off with a full tank-Hct 43- so we had a large safety factor and hadn't used much of it.

As I wrote the brief Op Note I put down an Estimated Blood Loss of 100cc and called to the anesthesiologist behind the screen, asking how much fluid she'd gotten. We had four anesthesiologists who did all our neuro cases, and I would have let any one of them put my family to sleep, so this was just a formality. The voice that answered back wasn't one I knew, and when I looked up there was some anesthesia resident I'd never seen before, telling me my patient had gotten 1500cc. of normal saline, oh, and by the way, 250 cc. of serum albumin. Serum is blood plasma; albumin is the major protein component of human blood.

I try not to scream "motherfucker" very often in the OR, as it has a negative effect on the team's overall morale, but it seems there are certain times nothing else will do. When some of the smoke cleared, I learned that the resident assigned to the case bailed just as we started closing because she's gotten a telephone message that her child was ill, and the current bozo had come in as her relief. The staff anesthesiologist- one of my four horsemen-hadn't clued this numbskull in on the 'no blood" policy before going next door to help intubate my partner's patient. Why should he have, since the operation was almost over, we were closing and hadn't lost any blood and Maria's vital signs were steady as a rock?

Nonetheless, this clown had decided he was bored and a little albumin probably wouldn't hurt her, so without asking me or the responsible anesthesiologist he'd hung a bottle. He's extraordinarily lucky I didn't shove that bottle right up his butt.

So now we-I- have violated the only request this lady, who also trusted me with her life, had made.

"Please don't give me any blood." Peachy keen.

Four hours later in the ICU, when she was awake and completely intact, I told her and her husband exactly what happened. I didn't go through all the precautions we'd taken, nor name the resident I would like to have killed, but I did make sure she knew I thought this was a terrible mistake, and one for which I ultimately had the blame. I think it may have helped that my old buddy Delbert was in the room. Maria listened, looked first at her husband, then at Delbert before telling me it was OK. She said it wasn't my fault and it wasn't her fault and she was just happy to be alive and intact. She smiled as she said, "No more blood, OK?"

I left the room with old Delbert in tow, and sat down over coffee with Maria's chart, just shaking my head. Delbert said, "Don't sweat it doc- you do good work. But, if I were you and this hospital, I'd probably make sure there are no charges for serum albumin on her bill. Do you get my meaning?"

I said," Fuck me."

CHAPTER NINE

Risky Business

I believe the most difficult forms of pathology a neurosurgeon treats operatively are the vascular abnormalities known collectively as arterio-venous malformations, abbreviated as AVMs. These are congenital lesions that arise during the embryological development of the brain and its blood vessels. For reasons as yet poorly understood, in about 1 in 700 newborns there will be a focal area of the brain which does not develop normally and as a consequence the blood vessels destined to serve that area never undergo the appropriate maturation; specifically, the entire capillary system in the affected area is completely absent. This absence results in preservation of the very rudimentary vascular system in which there exist a tangle of direct, uninterrupted abnormal vessels connecting the arterial and venous systems. The consequences of this maldevelopment are frequently disastrous..

In the normal brain, the high resistance capillary system is interposed between the very high-pressure arteries and the extraordinarily low pressure venous system. The capillaries, which are the body's smallest vessels, are the only site oxygen and glucose can leave the blood and enter into brain tissue. These tiny high-resistance vessels effectively dissipate all the propelling force of the heart, so in normal brains the blood arriving at the veins after passage through the capillary system is basically propelled solely by the force of gravity. Consequently, the walls of the veins are genetically designed to be thin, weak and distensible, whereas the arterial walls by design are thick and muscular, capable of withstanding the powerful impulses generated by the contracting heart muscle.

Absence of the capillary system has two serious consequences: 1) blood that passes through this abnormal vascular network area might as well be going to the feet as far as brain cells are concerned, because without the capillaries, the brain tissue normally supplied by these vessels cannot access the blood's oxygen and glucose, and 2) the weak veins receiving this blood are exposed to a very high pump pressure which they are not genetically constructed to handle. A third factor comes into play after this "shunt" has been in place for years. Blood flow is completely passive-it will preferentially go through this low resistance, abnormal system, rather than be forced through one of the adjacent, high resistance capillary networks. This passivity means that blood is chronically shunted away from brain that needs its oxygen and into this closed abnormal loop.

Consequently, an AVM is a compact nest of abnormal vessels under high pressure located in scarred, poorly developed brain tissue and surrounded by normal brain that is not receiving its normal blood supply. These nests can be of any size, and generally extend from the surface (or cortex) of the brain down deep two to three inches to the walls of the water chambers, or ventricles, which contain cerebrospinal fluid. These malformations most commonly announce their presence by rupturing, jetting high-pressure arterial blood into the brain and /or the underlying ventricle. Since brain tissue is about the same consistency of Jello left out of the refrigerator overnight, it doesn't pose significant resistance to this arterial stream that cuts into it like a knife into butter. In some patients, a sufficiently large clot will form within the brain itself stopping the hemorrhage; when this occurs, the patient may live until another bleed comes along, unless the clot is so big that its pressure threatens other functional areas. However, brain damaged by the hemorrhage isn't going to regrow and the nasty vascular nest isn't going away unless or until some befuddled surgeon decides to remove it.

Unlike tumors and aneurysms, each individual AVM is unique; unique in size, location, feeding vessels, draining veins, with perhaps an adjacent clot, or an aneurysm on one or more of its arteries. Unlike tumors and aneurysms, these explosive malformations can be located anywhere in the brain or, for that matter, in the spinal cord. To make matters worse, they are fragile, and unpredictable. Until Professor Yasargil developed a systematic technique of attacking them in the early 1970s, the only practical way to remove an AVM was to whack out a big surrounding chunk of normal brain along with the malformation, with the hope the patient could live with the neurological consequences. AVMs were a neurosurgeon's worst nightmare, and the bigger, the badder.

At our institution, we started cautiously being more aggressive with these fickle creatures after I returned from the Army, but it wasn't until I was joined by my partner Henry Baylor in 1983 that we evolved a consistent hard-nosed surgical approach to everyone we saw. Working together or spelling each other in the surgeon's chair, we educated one another in Yasargil's techniques for carefully isolating the nest from normal brain, of step-wise strangling every bit of their blood supply, of carefully chasing them down into the ventricles and then, once they were absolutely dead, gently removing the mass. But we learned to considerable dismay that often it wasn't over even then. Frequently the normal brain around the AVM, which ironically was now getting the blood supply it had been denied since it had been formed, would start to swell malignantly, with multiple bleeding points erupting in normal brain tissue. This complication required further patient gentle dissection, endless punctate coagulation and the aggressive use of tiny clips to seal off the most fragile vessels.

The surgical procedures themselves were of long duration, used lots of blood, and left many patients at least temporarily the worse for having the operation. The AVM may have been gone, but the price, all too often, was very dear. Operating on AVMs will teach a surgeon a lot of lessons: about neurosurgery, about taking care of sick people, about his colleagues, and mostly about himself.

In 1987, during the Christmas Holidays, I was sitting in my office when I got a call from an ER doc I played racquet ball with on week-ends. He had a patient for me, a psychiatrist who practiced at his hospital and had just been diagnosed with an AVM. He didn't know much about AVMs (or psychiatrists, it turned out), but he'd seen her studies and said, direct quote," This is a real bitch." I set her up to drop by the office the next day, which happened to be Christmas Eve, after checking to be sure Henry was going to be around. We saw her along with her partner that following afternoon.

Carole Lorris, who'd just turned fifty, had been complaining of horrible headaches for a couple of months before her partner, an ER nurse, in desperation put her stethoscope on the shrink's head. To everyone's surprise, she could hear a loud bruit, the sawmill sound (ZZHH-zzhh) blood makes when there's a lot of it moving with turbulent flow. The sound spooked them both. A CT scan and then an angiogram followed, after which their local neurosurgeon suggested she just live with it. No chance- the nurse talked to my racquet ball buddy, and here they were.

The AVM was massive. It occupied the back half of the right side of her brain and the multiple arteries supplying it were the size of Number 2 pencils. There was so much blood going to the damn thing that the arteriogram dye couldn't fill all the vessels, but every possible artery that could even conceivably pump blood to the lesion was doing so, to include arteries that normally supplied the scalp and skull.

The AVM was a monster, and the only good news was that it hadn't bled, meaning there was no big rush to take it out.

Henry and I had been fooling around with the concept of doing some preliminary things to the bigger AVMs before operating on them, things like injecting Crazy Glue into the feeding vessels to reduce the flow, and a neuro-radiologist working with us who had independently developed a technique of squirting small Teflon particles through a catheter into the feeding arteries as a means to block them off prior to surgery, but we'd not tackled something this big, so whatever we did was going to be risky business . We were upfront about that with Carole our prospective patient and her partner Grace.

Carole was adamant about getting rid of this thing, regardless of the risk. while Grace admittedly was a little less enthusiastic about the prospect. Because of her psychiatry practice, Carole needed about three months lead time to get her patients all referred to other therapists so we agreed on a tentative date in mid-March to start the preliminaries. Henry and I figured we'd have Phil Phillips, our neuro-radiologist with the Teflon, hammer the beast two or three times over a ten day period before we took Carole to the OR. Whether we injected the AVM with Crazy Glue before taking it out would depend on what we saw. We also arranged for Carole to bank a couple of units of her own blood prior to the procedure. As I mentioned, the only good thing about this situation was that we had time on our side, because Carole had not yet had a hemorrhage.

On a Thursday in early February, I was finishing a spine case in a small operating room when Henry walked in with the bad news. Carole had bled big time about eight that morning while doing her daily sit-ups She was now in a med-evac helicopter headed for our ER. The paramedic on board had intubated her when she'd stopped breathing; she still had a pulse, but that was about all.

It turned out that this Life Flight helicopter had a contractual arrangement with a hospital competitor across town. Consequently, the paramedics had planned to take Carole there, until Grace made them call our hospital, at which point one of our very best ever residents, Tim Adams, got on the horn with the pilot. The recording of that brief conversation is priceless: Tim advised the helo driver Carole was our patient and more importantly, that we were the only place where she had a chance of staying alive. When that didn't seem to impress the pilot, Tim promised that he personally would file manslaughter charges against the guy if they went elsewhere and Carole died. Talk about balls.

When I met Carole in the ER she was pretty close to dead; both pupils were dilated, she had a faint heartbeat, very low blood pressure and nothing else. As far as we could tell, her brain wasn't functioning. Henry was upstairs getting things ready, but the only operating room available was the ophthalmology room where there hadn't been a sick patient or a blood transfusion since the hospital opened in 1952. It was what we had, so up we went- five docs, three nurses, a respiratory therapist and Carole, all jammed in a tiny elevator.

In the OR, we turned Carole on her side, shaved her head and poured betadine over her scalp. Henry started with a huge horseshoe shaped incision that peeled down the back half of her scalp on the right. While we were drilling holes in her skull, the blood bank- which usually couldn't find its ass with both hands and a road map- came up with the one unit of her blood that had been banked the previous week and started working on a massive transfusion protocol to get more. By the time we got the big skull flap off, anesthesia had three big bore IVs in place and was pouring crystalloid in as fast as it would go. I still figured we basically had no chance.

It was Henry, Marissa Newman, our chief resident, and me. When we exposed Carole's dura mater it was so tight as to be almost bursting. One small nick with the knife and clot literally shot out, along with a belch of dead brain, all followed by fresh pulsating bright red arterial blood. Henry got most of it vacuumed up with a huge suction tube called appropriately a tonsil sucker, but then the real hemorrhage started. We put two more tonsils in the wound just to keep up. Carole's blood pressure was about 40 over nothing during this time, but the way she was bleeding I would have sworn it was three times that high.

All of the things a neurosurgeon would normally do to stop hemorrhage were completely worthless and all of our usual equipment was far too delicate to have any effect. It was like trying to stop a fire hose with a band-aid. Realizing we would never get the malformation itself to stop bleeding, we targeted the large vessels feeding it. I put my hand down into the brain itself to try to locate the large arteries and veins at the malformation's base. Every time I'd find one of these hoses, Henry would put a vascular clamp down at the approximate spot and I'd pinch off the vessel, usually producing a new fountain of blood from the free end of the freshly opened artery or vein before he could come back with a second clip. Marissa had a sucker in each hand, trying her best to keep up as we went around the circumference of the AVM pinching and clamping like two madmen.

The suctions roar when they're dealing with massive blood loss and the OR soon comes to smell like a butcher's shop. The nurses and anesthesiologists are yelling back and forth and there's absolutely nothing you can do to make any of it stop. And then, if you're very lucky, suddenly- literally within seconds- the suctions go silent... because the hemorrhage is over. Everyone who's been screaming at the top of their lungs looks embarrassed and shuts up. For a moment I thought the patient's heart had stopped, but Gary Archer, our laconic chief anesthesiologist, who never cursed, screamed: "For Christ's sake, have you finally stopped the bleeding?" And in fact, we had. Henry lifted what looked like a placenta out of the cavity we'd made, and the excitement was over.

It took another two hours to clean up the brain, coagulate the little feeders, wash all the open ventricular system out and cover the raw surfaces with a hemostatic gauze layer. Because we knew Carole was going to swell, Henry closed her dura over the huge hole in her brain (trust me, there was lots of room) but left the skull flap off to be replaced anther day if Carole survived. He put a couple of drains below the skin flap before Marissa and another resident closed the scalp in layers. We'd given Carole 27 units of blood, roughly three times the normal blood volume of a healthy human. Over the next day she'd get four more units.

Carole was unconscious for almost three days before gradually beginning to come around. Going to in- patient rehab a month later, she had an expressive aphasia (go figure), a dense left hemiparesis, and a complete field cut on the left. The visual field defect was permanent, but when we brought her back to replace the skull flap at six months post-bleed, her speech was fluent and her lower extremity strength was almost normal. Throughout the following year she fought for her recovery like a caged tiger, and on every clinic visit I could see she was stubbornly getting better.

Carole returned to her psychiatry practice 15 months after her hemorrhage with a stiff gait and a weak left arm. She remained in active practice for another eleven years until her death from a myocardial infarction. Carole Lorris was one tough lady.

In the late 1980s, these kinds of 'miraculous save' stories were being reported or talked about with increasing frequency as selected surgeons in American, Canada and Europe began to apply the principles of microvascular surgery first developed in Switzerland by Gazi Yasargil a decade and a half earlier. In Phoenix, Robert Spetzler was busy collecting the biggest AVM patient population in the world, while Roberto Heros at Harvard was critically analyzing his own and other surgeons' results, sorting out technical procedures that were successful from others that weren't. Meanwhile, the use of focused stereotaxic radiation was being popularized by the Stockholm group and endovascular embolization, initially reported in Russia but actually birthed by a group of talented

French neuroradiologists, was quickly coming to have a role in decreasing the vascular supply and therefore the risk of removing AVMs. But the ultimate responsibility for complete AVM elimination remained with neurosurgeons, and desperate patients, now empowered by the internet, began to travel for their definitive care.

In early 1988, we were contacted by an evangelical church group that supported a mission out-reach in Bangkok Thailand. There they had identified a 17-year-old young man who had suffered multiple bleeds from a large AVM that the Thais neurosurgeons were certain was inoperable." Inoperability" is, for better or worse, in the eye of the beholder, and when members of the church brought some of his images for us to review, Henry and I both independently felt this thing could be removed...probably. It was in a relatively unique location, deep in the crevasse that separates the brain's two hemispheres. The bad news- the exposure would be difficult and the most complicated, dangerous part of the operation would be done down in a deep dark hole. The good news- if there was any-was that the brain tissue around the malformation wasn't "eloquent", meaning not directly responsible for any major neurological functions. So, if we could manage to get the thing out without sacrificing any blood supply to the normal brain, in theory at least the kid should be all right. After a long discussion, we gave the church group a qualified "yes, we can do it."

There was more than a little hair on this situation. Since the church would be funding the entire ball of wax, they needed a special financial deal with our hospital. Despite wanting to be of help, the hospital powers-that-be had a lot of experience with our AVM patients, and knew up front there was no way we could predict how long the operation would take, how much blood we'd need, how long the patient would need ICU care, etc. Consequently, they were more than a little leery of making any bargains. In the administration's defense, Metro Memorial Hospital's responsibility was to the taxpayers of our county, not to a kid with a weird disease whose folks owned a kite shop in Bangkok. However, the hospital also was very sensitive to the salutary effects of good publicity.

The tie-breaker turned out to be CBS News, which was shopping around for a big hospital to feature on its new show "48 Hours". The network was entranced by the story, the proposed operation and its attendant drama. So, long story short, on a chilly January morning Henry and I, with Dan Rather peering over our shoulders, took young Maylai Pangich to the OR for what turned out to be a bona fide blood bath.

I'm still not exactly sure where the train left the track. At about nine hours after we started (say 7 PM) I thought we were almost completely around the AVM and not too far from delivering it, intact, from its bed. We'd lost 6-7 units of blood, but Gary and Lee Boots were right on top of that and thus far there was no evidence of any of the clotting problems that can accompany large volume transfusions. The brain still looked healthy, and even down in the depths around the malformation there was a nice demarcation between "good" and "bad" brain. Henry and I were trading off every couple of hours under the scope so the whole situation was in a lot better shape than I would have predicted. The TV people were professional, accomplished and very careful to stay out of the way. After the first hour or so, they were just part of the furniture.

The problem started at the very back part of the exposure in the deepest part of the wound- just a little "troublesome" bleeding that didn't respond to the usual tricks but didn't actually get worse right away. I packed it off with a cotton pledget, which seemed to slow things down for a minute or two, but then I noticed the brain was getting "tight", meaning it was swelling within the skull. There are a few reasons that can happen, but when you've run your checklist and haven't found the cause, especially if you're operating in or around the ventricles (water chambers), you have to figure that whatever you're operating on is bleeding into the ventricles and filling up the brain.

Maylai's AVM was situated right on top of three of the four ventricles, and when I opened into them they were chock full of clotted blood. As I evacuated clot, the ventricles filled right back up with bright red arterial blood from a source neither of us could identify. After about an hour of this, the bleeding intensified, and from then on it was a dogfight. Lots of noise, overwhelming smell of blood, people running around, suckers plugging up – and all the while you're straining to keep your hands steady and still make miniscule, important movements with slender instruments in a small hole five inches deep in a boy's brain.

By four o'clock in the morning Maylai had received twenty units of blood and was still bleeding from a deep source we couldn't identify. If I could have reached my hand down into the wound, I probably could have stopped the hemorrhage, but the hole was far too deep and only barely big enough for one finger, so I didn't even try. The blood bank had run out of cross-matched blood, so now Maylai was getting what's called "universal donor" or O negative blood and we was beginning to have trouble with the blood not clotting. His 17-year-old heart was fine and his kidneys were making good urine, but the brain was looking bruised and soggy. I figured we had maybe another thirty minutes. I could see what appeared to be a serious bleeding point almost out of reach of our instruments, but when I stretched for it, my forceps were shaking so badly, they ended up in the walls of the ventricle. I asked Henry to take a shot- we both knew I meant last shot- so he sat down, threaded a clip right into the bottom of the hole and turned it loose. Just like that, the hemorrhage stopped.

When the bleeding stops because you've actually taken an AVM out, there's a sense of success, finality, victory, something. On the other hand, when the bleeding stops because you've stuck a clip on something you can't even identify, you're afraid to breathe. So we sat there for another hour, waiting for the next explosion. We made sure Maylai's blood level was normal, his electrolytes all in the boxes, blood pressure just right, his EKG perfect and even did a chest x-ray, which was normal. So, what's next?

To be a good surgeon, it helps to be tough, but more importantly, you'd better avoid being stupid. Over that twenty-three hours, Maylai, Henry and I had had about all the surgery we could individually stand. It's galling to quit when you haven't accomplished what you came to do, but it's worse to allow your pride to subject a patient to a risk you don't understand and aren't even certain you could overcome if you did. So, reluctantly, we bailed.

Lining the cavity of the resection cavity in Maylai's brain with hemostatic gauze backed up with cotton, we made certain that the wound was completely dry-"dusty"- then closed his head. Back in the ICU, our troops rigidly controlled his blood pressure until the afternoon, then we went to angiography to see what was what. As might have been expected, we'd inadvertently cut across the very far corner of the AVM; we saw about ½ cm. of malformation that was amputated by Henry's clip. A month later, we took Maylai back to the OR to take out the cotton, the gauze, the clip and the small nubbin of AVM.

It pays to be seventeen. With all his bills paid, the hospital happy and CBS elated about "48 Hours", Maylai went back to Bangkok six weeks after his initial operation. The boy was a celebrity, and the family's kite shop prospered. He's now the proprietor, and up until a couple of years ago, we traded Christmas cards regular as clockwork. The 48 Hours segment was first shown late that same January, and I haven't been able to watch it since. It's been 29 years.

AVM surgery carries a lot of potential for disaster beyond simple exsanguination. The good AVM surgeons, like the guys mentioned above, always have their heads on a swivel, continuously on the lookout for any one of the myriad of things that, because they can go wrong, will go wrong. That's only one of the reasons that the medical centers that do this surgery best are institutions that always have a lot of eyes on the ball. AVM surgery is no place for solo operators.

About ten years ago I was asked to see an AVM patient who, we learned in getting the routine details, was about six months after a surgical procedure at the hands of another neurosurgeon in our region of the country. I knew the guy slightly, thought he was a pretty fair general neurosurgeon, but was surprised he'd elected to take on this type case. The circumstances around the young patient's clinical condition were murky; I began to smell a rat when his mother insisted that the family's attorney attend the consultation.

The kid was 26, in prior good health, previously employed at a Wal-Mart in a little West Texas town a hundred or so miles from our medical center. The recent onset of headaches, coupled with some poorly-described difficulty with his vision had prompted his LMD (local medical doctor) to obtain a CT scan and then a hurried consultation with a neurosurgery group in the regional population center, a town of about 50,000 residents. By the luck of the draw, Patrick, our patient, was scheduled to see the newest member of the group, a young man who'd been out of his residency a couple of years. This practice was big and booming. It made a lot of money doing disc and spine surgery but probably wasn't the place you'd choose to have your head operated on unless it was a real emergency. Definitely not the Massachusetts General.

On the day of Patrick's appointment, our chief resident, whose name was Mark, went into see and examine Patrick first. There was a little kerfuffle from Mom and the attorney about whom the resident was and what he was going to do. Linda, our nurse, requested I stick my head in the door, so I did, explaining that our residents saw every patient first and that this policy was outlined in large print in the patient information brochure they'd received and autographed when they came in the clinic door. Things quieted down and about twenty minutes later, Mark came back to brief me on what he'd learned.

In the meanwhile, I'd been looking at Patrick's images. The AVM shown in the angiogram was small, a tight group of vessels about ¾ inch in diameter located on the inner surface of Patrick's right temporal lobe. To expose it surgically would be a little bit of a stretch without going through the lobe itself, but it's generally bad neurosurgical form to violate good brain if you don't absolutely have to, and I figured that in a "relaxed" brain (one that's not swollen or inflamed) we'd definitely be able to sneak up on this puppy without opening the temporal lobe. As a plus, there were only two arteries of any size feeding the AVM, and by approaching it the long way around, we'd encounter both of them long before they entered the brain, a sequence that would allow us to basically disarm the thing before we ever saw it. I was pretty excited about what appeared to be an elegant surgical solution, but when I saw the look on Mark's face my enthusiasm faded.

He said, "Boss, this is pretty miserable. Apparently, the AVM is gone, but the kid's been wrecked. There's something bad wrong with his brain; he's got a visual problem, but the big thing seems to be that he remembers absolutely nothing, barely recognizes even his parents and has to be led from place to place, even to the bathroom. He can't recognize any objects; I gave him my reflex hammer and he put it right in his mouth, which his mother says is his go-to move with everything. His speech, when you can get anything out of him, is slow and kind of flight-of-ideas. He can't or won't really cooperate with a neurological exam, but I don't find any focal weakness or sensory loss. He walks OK, but like I said, they have to basically lead him around. And here's the kicker; he's got surgical scars on both sides of his head. Mom says the surgeon had to operate on both sides to get the AVM out."

As I trooped back with Mark to the exam room, somewhere in the back of my head a faint bell was ringing. After looking Patrick over and listening to his mother, the bell got a lot louder. Mom told us that, about four hours into her son's surgery, the surgeon had come out to the waiting room to tell the family that he'd not been able to remove the AVM successfully from his original approach through the right temporal lobe, so he was going to make a second incision on the left to expose and remove it from that direction. After another three hours or so, he'd returned to say that plan had been successful, but because of the lengthy surgery, Patrick would probably be "a little slow to come around."

In fact, the kid apparently emerged from anesthesia pretty quickly, but had been devastated neurologically ever since. The neurosurgeon had finally suggested a neurology consult. Once the neurologist had taken a close look, he then sent them to us in the big city. Mom said he'd mentioned something about "Clover Bucky" disease several times. Now my faint bell was tolling like Big Ben.

In the late 1930s a neurologist in Chicago named Henrich Kluver was experimenting with mescaline as an anti-seizure medication and convinced Paul Bucy, a prominent neurosurgeon, to help him with his studies by removing both temporal lobes in a group of rhesus monkeys. The mescaline part of the experiment flamed out, but post-operatively the monkeys developed a consistent weird behavior disorder that centered around inability to recognize objects, an inability to learn tasks which ultimately proved to be a memory disorder and a profound docility. Some of the monkeys were hypersexual, others ate everything in sight while some seemed only able to recognize familiar objects by putting them in their mouths. The two physicians reported their results in the medical literature and the constellation of symptoms quickly became known as the Kluver-Bucy syndrome. Subsequently, several adult patients having had both temporal lobes injured or destroyed by infection, trauma or surgery were found to have the same symptoms complex; in 1966 one of these patients had been presented at Washington University School of Medicine Neurology Grand Rounds. I can't remember the nature of his injury, but his pitiful disability made a lasting impression on this sophomore medical student.

What had happened was pretty obvious. Confused about which temporal lobe was involved, the neurosurgeon had initially operated on the incorrect side. After plowing through the normal temporal lobe for two hours, he'd recognized his mistake, turned the kid over and gone in from the opposite side. His choice of approach- directly through the brain itself – had destroyed this temporal lobe as well, although he had managed to find and excise the AVM. He had recommended that Patrick and his family come to see us "to see if any thing else could be done" The attorney came along to make certain all his ducks were in a row for the malpractice case, which had already been filed.

One of the cardinal rules of a good surgeon is to be keenly aware of your own limitations. Another is to always have the patient's best interest at heart. Neurosurgery, by its very nature is a risky business, so it's not impossible to make four critical mistakes in any one operation, but when it happens, it will be in a tough case, like an AVM. If you operate on the wrong side of the head (1) through an inappropriate route (2) and then compound it by mindlessly doing the same thing on the opposite side (3), you've firmly verified your dismal lack of judgment in accepting the case in the first place (4). This last error, an egregious violation of the Good Surgeon's Rules, paves the way for most surgical disasters.

CHAPTER TEN

The Professor

A concern about end of life issues has been a large part of my professional career since early on in my training (*see Chapter 11- measles*) and in fact, was the topic of a two-hour discussion with my wife Patricia on our first date. Patricia is a trauma / critical care surgeon at, one of our country's largest and most famous trauma centers, as well as a medical ethicist whose opinions on issues such as this radiate amazing clarity. We've learned a lot from each other over the thirty-plus years we've been taking care of critically ill patients together, and more often than not I've been the student.

A large amount of the recent controversy about euthanasia and physician-assisted suicide has been complicated and perhaps even confounded by debate of issues such as "the slippery slope ", "unintended effect", "passive versus active measures", etc. whereas there has been insufficient focus on the concept of a "good death", which is, in fact, the meaning of the word euthanasia. I believe not enough emphasis has been placed on identifying the components of a "good death" and specifying who is responsible for making that determination. So, let me tell you about a patient we took care of some fifteen years ago.

John Ashton was a world-famous physicist who played a seminal role during the Space Shuttle Project at NASA and then became the chairman of the physics department at the University of Texas at Dallas.

He was a widower with three adult children, multiple grandkids and an adoring retinue of faculty members and graduate students. Dr. Ashton was eighty-two years of age, in excellent health and a rabid Dallas Cowboys fan.

He lived on the UTD campus and part of his good health he attributed to his daily early morning bicycle rides around the campus, during which he passed directly in front of the University's fire station. On pleasant mornings, like we sometimes have in late September, the on-call fire/rescue crew, sitting out on the station's front porch, would exchange greetings with the Doc as he peddled past.

On this September Monday morning, for reasons still not explained, as Dr. Ashton passed the station the front brakes of his mountain bike suddenly and unexpectedly locked up. He went down directly over the handlebars in full view of the fire fighters, who naturally rushed to the rescue. John's bike helmet had a bad scrape on the brim above his forehead and he had only a small laceration on his chin, but quickly the fire guys understood that although his eyes were open, his lips were moving, and he was taking short breaths, the Doc couldn't move his extremities. As John's breathing quickly became more labored, they realized he had some kind of brain or spine injury, and someone brought the ER Trauma kit from the ambulance. Dr. Ashton was unconscious by the time they slipped an oral airway in to ventilate him with a bag, but he rapidly regained consciousness, shaking his head appropriately to every question he was asked. The fire team put him in a hard cervical collar on a back board, then brought him through our ER's doors about twenty minutes later.

When I first saw John, he'd been intubated after being given a short-acting muscle relaxant and anesthetic combination, had two big bore IVs and a Foley catheter in place and had just had the first images made of his cervical spine. He was completely with it, but other than a weak shoulder shrug, Dr. Ashton had no motor or sensory function below his clavicles. He was what medicine terms "complete", a complete quadriplegic at a "high level", meaning that almost none of his spinal cord was functioning. His images showed that he had suffered a "Hangman's Fracture".

This is a relatively complicated fracture -dislocation of the second and third cervical vertebrae in which the bony ring of C2 is torn apart with the front being displaced anteriorly along with C1 and the skull while the back or posterior half remains in place atop C3 and the rest of the spine. This fracture- dislocation effectively crushes the spinal cord at the C2-3 level; its well-deserved gruesome name stems from the results of judicial hangings in which, contrary to lore, the hangman's knot is placed beneath the hangee's chin.

Fatalities due to these fractures are secondary to asphyxiation, as the muscles of respiration are paralyzed by the cord's injury. Surprisingly, not all of these fractures are fatal and some even have no cord injury if the lucky patient has only the fracture without the ensuing dislocation. Generally, the dislocation is relatively easy to reduce (put back into place). However, as a rule, Hangman's Fractures are an immediate death sentence, except when they happen right in front of a fire/ rescue crew.

We put Dr. Ashton in a traction device that consists of a large ring which embraces the head and is anchored to it by two pins which penetrate the skull bone just above each ear. Sounds ugly, but with the help of a little local anesthetic at the puncture sites, the application is pretty much painless; with proper maintenance these tongs will carry a lot of weight for a protracted time period. John's fracture was quickly reduced with a small amount of traction and proved easy to maintain in proper alignment, but none of that made his spinal cord work any better.

Once the professor was as stable as he was going to get, we sent him down to Radiology for a full set of images, to include CT and MR. CT scanning is the absolute cat's ass in looking for bony abnormalities while MR shows the spinal cord in almost unbelievable detail, so when the two studies were completed at the end of the day, we had a comprehensive picture of Dr. Ashton's anatomy. It wasn't pretty. The fracture itself, a garden variety break of the C3 pedicles with an added teardrop fracture of the body of C2, didn't mean much. The spinal cord on the other hand looked like it had been hammered from C2 down to C4. There was some patchy blood in the substance of the cord, which is not a good sign, and we could already see severe swelling that tailed off around C5. The cord wasn't physically cut in two, but it might as well have been.

A physician can, and should, put off giving his patient bad news until all the information is in, but once the images are done, it's time to lay it all out, especially with someone like Dr. Ashton. So, I told him the facts. The outlook was pretty bleak, although he might regain some function when the swelling, or edema, of the cord went down and the blood started to clear itself, all of which would probably be around the end of the week. In the meanwhile, we'd be giving him some steroids which might help with the edema, keeping him hydrated and making sure he wasn't in pain. Communication was going to be a problem, because of this big endotracheal tube that extended from his lips down into his trachea and was attached to the mechanical ventilator keeping him alive; he could nod his head or shake it and the nurses would teach him a simple code so that he could signal with his eyes, but John wouldn't be able to speak, which would become more important as his family began to arrive the following day. When I asked him if he understood, his gaze never wavered as he nodded his head.

How much of what I said was true? Almost, but not quite all. While it's a fact that the immediate visible effects of severe spinal cord injuries do start to recede on imaging studies around four days post-injury, that recession only rarely signals a significant return of neurological function, especially in a cord injured this badly and at this high a level. For Dr. A to regain enough function just to breath on his own would mean he'd have to improve from a C2 to a C4 or C5 level of function; even then he'd have no use of his arms, much less his legs. The odds of even that degree of improvement in an 82-year-old were probably not zero but awfully close; I'd certainly never seen or heard of it. But hope, even a just little hope, is important for both patients and doctors, and as long as that faint possibility existed, we all needed to acknowledge it. It would help everyone get through the next week.

The professor's kids came in the next day, all three of them, and they were something to behold. Two men and a woman in their forties and fifties; bright, courteous, compassionate, understanding, and above all, very loving towards their dad. You could see in his face, bunged up with abrasions and twisted by tape, the pride for this miracle he and his wife had birthed. They lit up the ICU like fresh air, and it broke my heart that I had only bad news to tell them. But this wasn't a one-way street.

After I'd been through everything, including showing them the images and demonstrating on a plastic model of the spine how it all came down, they started with their own questions.

How much can he feel? Why is he being turned so often? Is he in pain? Is he hungry or thirsty? Can we get that tube out of his mouth? Assuming the very best, what kind of recovery- what could he do? These and more; not asked in an accusatory manner, but trying to understand what was going on with one of the most important persons in each of their lives. The answers were simple but not easy, and they pinned me to the wall when I started talking about the cord swelling and the possibility the professor would improve if and when it began to recede.

'Was that a real possibility?'

'Yes.'

'Had I ever seen people hurt this bad get better?'

'No.'

'How long can he live like this?'

'Until he gets an infection we can't treat.'

'Would you let your dad live like this?'

'Not a chance.'

That's when they brought out Dr. Ashton's living will. Each of them had a copy, each had discussed it with their father and all three were absolutely certain this wasn't living as the professor defined it. We could either honor it or they'd take him some place that would. Full stop.

Dealing with people like the Ashton family is a small but important part of what makes medicine the greatest career in the world. Here's a family whose heart is broken by the most horrible injury to their father that I can imagine and whose sole thoughts are for him, for his suffering and for what he -not they-wants.

So, we talked some more and made a plan. I believed it was only right that we ride this out until it was clear it wasn't going anywhere good, and by everything I knew, that meant the week-end. I'd said that to the professor when he came in, to his family now, and that was the only medical demand I 'd make, other than we have the latitude to make certain he didn't suffer.

They said the only thing Dr. Ashton loved almost as much as his family and physics was the Cowboys, so we checked and fortunately they didn't have an off week that Sunday. I think if they had been scheduled to be off I would have asked them to televise a scrimmage because this was important to a man who was going to die that afternoon. Then I made sure we could get a big TV set in the ICU room, because usually there's no need for one, and finally- the most important step- we brought the ICU nurses into the consultation room to explain what was going to happen.

In the armed services it's common knowledge that the backbone of every unit isn't its officers nor its grunts, but rather the non-commissioned officers, the sergeants, chiefs, petty officers and gunnies who make the whole damn thing run. In an ICU, that's the nurses. They are the spirit of the unit; they make things happen and not happen, go fast or slow, be good or bad, so if they're not with you, you're screwed and deserve it. They know the patients, not just their diseases, and the families and their conflicts and hang-ups and emotions. They're the life-blood of every ICU, so if you plan to do something a little hinky, they better be onboard.

And they were. There're not many surprises in the pressure cooker of a Trauma ICU. Most everybody knows what's going on, almost before it happens, so the fact we'd decided to let Dr. A die wasn't a secret for very long. However, it was important to hold that information close for four days, which was no cakewalk. There's a necessary tension between care-givers and administrators in every health care institution. I'd be among the first to admit that the suits have an important role in keeping the lights on and the trash picked up, but this kind of thing was way out of their ball park and needed to stay there.

And this in an environment notorious for the lightning speed and stunning exaggeration of its grapevine. If a doc and a nurse have a thirty second conversation at a scrub sink at 0800, by noon everyone in surgery thinks they're sleeping together and by 1600 she's pregnant with twins and he's left his wife and three kids. So, four days is a long time, but we did it.

By Saturday, the professor had showed no improvement and was in increasing pain to judge by his morphine doses. His chest film made it look like pneumonia wasn't far off, but the ventilator was keeping him well oxygenated, and his children and a few grandchildren were with him at all times when he was awake. An adult stayed in the room even as he slept so that he'd not awaken alone. We got a quick MR that morning to check his cord, and as expected, the edema was less and there was no more evidence of hemorrhage so that faint hope was essentially gone.

After examining him and looking at the films I told him any improvement seemed less and less likely, so if he wanted for us to continue to be aggressive, there were a couple of things we needed to get done. One was a tracheostomy, which would allow us to get that tube out of his mouth and replace it with one inserted in a small surgical incision in his neck; the other was a gastrostomy, placement of a small tube through the skin of his abdomen and into his stomach through which he could get nutrition. Both of these things were pretty minor and could easily be done in one morning.

After I went through my explanation, the side of his mouth that I could see smiled, and he shook his head from side to side. His daughter was sitting with him; she said, "Dad's ready to have this over with."

I looked back at Dr. Ashton. "Sir, do you want to be done with these supportive treatments, the tubes, ventilator, IVs? Do you want us to withdraw care?"

Another half-smile and a big nod.

I sighed, then smiled as well. "Well, we need to watch those Cowboys tomorrow, correct?" Another smile.

Later I spoke with the Professor's two sons in the consultation room, his daughter still staying with her dad. I told them about the plan the Trauma team and I had concocted on the fly the prior day. Our goal was to make this as painless as possible for him and then secondarily for everyone else. Practically that translated into taking the fear out of the process, and the ultimate anxiety of air hunger and any pain associated with removing the endotracheal tube completely away. None of us had ever done anything like this, at least that we'd admit to, but we all knew the final fatal pathway was oxygen deprivation, and that would happen without us doing anything other than disconnecting our patient from the ventilator. The family knew the tube was essential for the respirator

119

but wanted to say good-bye to Dad/ Granddad without it being there. Before the tube was out, we wanted instantaneous unconsciousness and no struggles, so we'd settled on a central nervous system depressant much like Valium, coupled with a big dose of morphine, and a muscle paralytic, the latter to prevent the involuntary muscle contractions that come when the muscles are running out of oxygen.

Surprisingly, when we came around to deciding who was going to give the drugs, there were a lot of volunteers. A bunch of folks had, over a very short time, come to care about this gentleman and his family and every one of his care-givers felt this was the right thing to do. Finally, we settled on a guy I'll call Dr. Bill, who was in charge of the Trauma team that had admitted Dr. Ashton and had remained responsible for taking care of everything but his neck since the get-go. Bill had not been a part of delivering that bad news day after day and thus had what was probably the most "normal" relationship with the Ashton family. When I explained our choice to the sons and daughter, they were on board.

Now only one person left to tell. With the family at the Professor's bedside that afternoon, I went through the entire song and dance one more time, reciting what had happened to his spinal cord, what we'd hoped would occur over the week, how the images were improved but he wasn't and what the outlook was for the future. I made him tell me again that he didn't want to go down that road, and then I explained our cobbled-together alternative. He nodded his way through my explanation, then gave me his half-smile one more time, closed his eyes and nodded again.

On Sunday, the Cowboys kept it close until the fourth quarter and then won going away. There was a little beer drunk in the second half that everybody including the nurses ignored and then, once it was over, the grandkids who were all crying gave Granddad a hug and left the room with their parents, all three of whom came back in a minute later. The three of them gathered around and talked to their dad for a while and then his daughter looked up at Bill with a brief nod. Standing behind the Professor's left shoulder, he pushed the first drug into the IV port then opened up the line to flush it.

The kids kept talking as their father's eyes closed and after about a minute Bill pushed the second syringe. One of the Trauma fellows disconnected the ventilator as a nurse turned it off, then deflated the cuff of the tube and gently pulled it out. Air trapped behind the cuff escaped in a sigh that startled the family, but the nurses quickly cleaned the excess tape off the professor's face and then got out of the way. Bill reached up to turn off the alarm of the EKG monitor and we all stepped back to watch the little green tracing gradually slow and then come to a stop.

A good death.

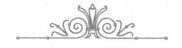

CHAPTER ELEVEN

Measles

In my first week of internship I landed on the Neurosurgery Service at Mr. Duke's Hospital under the tender mercies of Dr. Guy Odom and his impressive faculty and resident staff. On my very first call night, Dr. Odom and I developed a special relationship when one of his pre-op patients, naturally hospitalized the evening before surgery, asked me to call Dr. Odom at home with a few questions she'd forgotten to ask during her clinic visit. I don't remember exactly how I got Dr. Odom's number, and it didn't seem to me that 11:30 on Tuesday was all that late, but right after he answered and I identified myself, I came to the realization that there were several obligatory levels of communication interposed between intern and department chairman.

Fortunately, neither us held a grudge. He was such a charismatic surgeon and I was such a glutton for punishment that I tried to get in the OR every time he was operating. Dr. Odom always operated with two assistants, the chief resident and either an intern or a junior resident, so to get a spot at the table meant trading off with one of the junior residents on the service, more specifically, Dr. Steph Crockett. Steph, who later, when we were both at Walter Reed for a year, became a long-term friend, was a really interesting guy. He'd come back to Duke to complete his neurosurgery residency after serving 13 months as a Special Forces doc in Vietnam. He didn't say a hell of a lot. but when he talked it was straight-forward, thoughtful stuff, as to be differentiated from a lot of the bullshit that passed for advice to the interns.

About half way thru my six-week rotation, Dr. Odom admitted a young woman, 27 years of age, married with one kid, who had a large 3-4 cm. cerebello-pontine angle tumor. She'd been worked up elsewhere, then seen by Dr. Odom in his clinic and scheduled for surgery. After her admission on the evening prior to her operation I did her history and physical, got to know her and her family a little, drew her blood, then turned her over to Steph who would the first of two (junior-chief) residents to see her that night. Then Dr. Odom came in for his pre-op visit. After he talked with the patient we all tagged along over to his office where he looked again at her technitiem brain scan and her air study, then outlined his operative plan. This man was a master surgeon and one hell of a guy. In many important ways he was very much like his celebrated Canadian friend, Dr. Charles Drake, so if you were a wannabe neurosurgeon in 1969, any time you could spend with him was precious.

The next morning Steph and I alternated holding up the cerebellum with ribbon retractors while the big chief, using loupes and assisted by Dr Ray Tanaka on the monopolar cautery, took this meningioma out piece by piece in a little over four hours. Dr Odom was a meticulous surgeon, and from where I was draped over the patient's head, there didn't seem to be much blood loss. However, late in the case I saw the anesthesia resident (the staff was out to lunch in more ways than he knew) transfuse a single unit of red cells. I thought that was a little strange, but I'd already learned that interns on the Duke Neurosurgery Service weren't being paid for their opinions, so I kept my mouth shut.

Despite the two of us rookies jerking on her cerebellar hemisphere for what seemed like forever, this young woman awoke promptly from anesthesia with only a mild facial nerve paresis, called me by name in the recovery area, and was able to give her husband a big hug and a skewed kiss within about an hour of the last skin stitch. She was fine on check-out rounds that evening, but about six hours later she had a massive transfusion reaction, bled into her head, developed a consumptive coagulopathy and died early the next morning just after I came back for morning rounds.

The tragic young lady was the first of "my" patients to die. That, fact added to the unexpected nature of her death coupled with her young age, obvious good health and that she was a real person to me almost put me in a trance. We were on-call every other night, so the evening of her death Steph and I were padding out after evening rounds, and I was pretty far along the path to becoming a real zombie.

Finally, Dr. Crockett leaned across the table, grabbed my arm and acted like he was going to crawl down my scrub shirt. He said, "Listen - you better get your shit together; we're not treating the measles here." The physical nature of that confrontation dislodged my head from my lower GI tract, but throughout my subsequent career as both a teacher and a surgeon it's been his short powerful summary of the situation that's proven most important.

I certainly wasn't the first, nor would I be the last would-be neurosurgery resident to need a crash course in looking at death and destruction up close. That's a little paradoxical because a large percentage of our country's population will die or be devastated by diseases with important neurosurgical implications. That list is too long and familiar to recite, as are the complications of many of the treatments we provide, but when you sum them all up, as the man said, pretty soon you're talking some real numbers.

It's true that the rapidity of many of these illnesses rob patients of their individual identities early after disease onset and certainly well before a neurosurgeon ever darkens their door, but others lead to months and sometimes years of progressive, often painful neurological disability, cognitive and emotional decline and abject misery. So, the neurosurgical patient's dying trajectory, that is the time from LKW (last-known-well) to death, can and does vary from short and depersonalized to long and agonizing. More often than not, as neurosurgeons we're not only along for the ride but supposedly have something positive to contribute.

I want to share a few thoughts, not about the dying patient, but about that patient's neurosurgeon; what he or she may feel and how those feelings may affect the surgeon's personal and professional lives. The caveat should be obvious: this is just one surgeon's experience rather than a summary of broadly-held opinions or even a tentative suggestion about "how things ought to be." Despite having seen and discussed many of these issues with colleagues, friends and students over a long practice life, I'm all too cognizant that in the cauldron of a busy clinical practice sometimes it's hard to even stay in touch with your own emotions, much less be able to claim insight into those around you. So this is just me.

There's a lot of wisdom in the old adage, first said about human combat: "Those that speak don't know and those that know don't speak." However, I do believe that one can both know and speak a little about patient morbidity / mortality, and furthermore that we as physicians shortchange our patients, our students and ourselves by failing to make a conscious attempt to communicate more frequently and in more depth in the face of the inevitable mortality we encounter in clinical medicine.

For me, the misery of a patient's injury or death, especially if unexpected, releases a complex wave of emotions. I'm certain the components of that mixture are different for every surgeon, but personally, first and foremost is a sense of chilling defeat, almost regardless of the nature of the disease or injury. I interpret my job as making the patient better. Having actually been to medical school, I understand we're all going to die, but you don't have to do it while I'm taking care of you. So death equates with personal failure. It's not a vague emotion but a jolting stab of revolting personal inadequacy.

This is probably a reflection of the commitment all physicians make to do the "right thing", and our unwavering belief, despite copious examples to the contrary, that the right thing will always have beneficial consequences. While the term "sacred" has different meanings to different people, I believe most physicians would feel comfortable describing this commitment in that fashion. Consequently, when my patient is hurt or dying despite my best skills, insight and experience, it's a harsh reflection on the way I define myself. There are a couple of ways to deal with that harshness:

DENIAL

As my old friend Steph forcibly reminded me four decades ago, we're in a no-joke, high-stakes business. Many of the diseases we treat still refuse to surrender their horrible natural histories to the miracles of medicine and the technological advances of modern surgery. Even worse, these particular maladies continue to kill and cripple by attacking the very personal essences of our patients and ourselves. Facing that type of relentless opposition, sometimes just in order to keep coming to work every day you have to focus on the infrequent wins versus the ever-present losses. Nonetheless, just desperately pretending the outcome will be different doesn't make it so, either for the surgeon, the patient, or the family. Consequently, denial, as an operative strategy, doesn't have much to say for itself. While it may delay the psychological angst of facing the music, in an acute clinical setting denial can have negative practical effects by delaying or even preventing an intense search for techniques to ameliorate the situation.

Even in the most dire straits, a stiff dose of honesty followed by some creative out-of-the-box thinking is sometimes -although not very often-a "winner." The idea that "we'll just keep our fingers crossed" won't cut it here. As uncomfortable as it might be, an acute rational interpretation of a horrible clinical situation is crucial to identifying a potential solution if one exists.

This type of hard-nosed attitude is essential not only in the acute clinical setting but also in a more removed analysis of one's own work, where rude honesty plays an important role in a surgeon's self- awareness and ultimately his or her personal integrity. Unfortunately, intellectual dishonesty is not uncommon in medicine; even a cursory evaluation of much of medical reporting uncovers published success rates and morbidity / mortality figures right out of Grimm's Fairy Tales. That self-aggrandizing, self-deceit begins with conscious or sub-conscious manipulation of operative results, patient outcomes, etc. Although most of my career has focused on vascular disease (where this behavior has been endemic) it's especially common currently in the epidemic of spinal surgery that's swept the country over the past 15 years, and should be an absolute disqualifier for referrals, promotions and recognition.

ANGER

Anger is a natural, visceral and almost instantaneous response to personal insult or injury (such as the sense of personal failure), and its target can be external or internal. Anger's consequences are variable; in the OR, for example, if anger can be channeled and focused on the 'badness' - the AVM that won't stop bleeding, the tumor stubbornly attached to the optic chiasm or the disc fragment locked under the nerve root - anger can be an advantage to the surgeon, making him/her colder, harder, stronger; more intent and unwilling to settle for any outcome other than "the right thing."

Unfortunately, especially in the face of looming morbidity or mortality, anger represents a costly diversion from the real issue. I can hate the disease and what it's doing to my patient, and I can hate my own helplessness, but if I can't recognize the emotion for what it is and choke it off in a corner to be dealt with later, this anger can be irreversibly destructive. All of us that are old enough have seen the uniformly negative effects on everyone in range of a surgeon's temper tantrums which poison the atmosphere necessary for teamwork, destroy the sense of focus critical to operative efficiency and all too often scapegoat an innocent team member for what are often the surgeon's own inadequacies or the irreversible anatomical facts.

In the worst of situations, uncontrolled anger will emotionally distance the surgeon from his/ her patient and equally importantly from the patient's family. It's a cruel irony that extremely-ill patients and their families desperately crave the affection and approval of their physicians. They are exquisitely attuned to their surgeons' emotions and very vulnerable to mistaking anger as being directed at them, rather than their disease process.

Personally, I've found it impossible to be angry and simultaneously reach out in a meaningful way to patients and families in real pain. While I've never been completely able to abolish my initial angry reactions, I have learned to stifle their manifestations and their negative effects on my ability to communicate. That issue is definitely complicated when my anger is entangled with yet another problematic response - guilt.

GUILT

An introspective physician immersed in patient care can usually find multiple reasons to feel guilty during any given day. There are the patients you thoughtlessly made wait in your clinic, the family you shorted on time prior to operating on their loved one, the nurse/ intern/

colleague you may have barked at impatiently- the list is limited only by your selective memory. However, in dealing solely with issues of patient morbidity and mortality, I think there are two specific forms of self-recrimination that are important to recognize. I'll designate them as little guilt and big Guilt.

The first and fortunately most common form of guilt is a pervasive sense of self-recrimination experienced by many physicians as a result of patients dying in the natural course of their disease processes. This emotion I believe has more to do with an existential sorrow related to the inequity of death coupled with our inability to provide ultimate intervention than it does to a sense of personal culpability. In some situations, a tinge of guilty pleasure of having been temporarily "spared" may also creep in to play a minor role, always followed by the insight that 'temporarily' is the operative word. I think this type guilt is closely akin to the spontaneous anger I mentioned previously; it is emphatically different from the soul-searing self-hatred that attends surgeons' mistakes. Guilt "with a small g" is a vague sense of remorse which not infrequently will distance the physician from his / her patient. In some extreme situations, this emotion, which has been termed "disenchantment with the entire living -dying process," may even imperil the physician's willingness to continue in active practice. I confess this form of disembodied guilt is not a personally familiar emotion, so rather than discuss it farther; I'm going to turn to a different aspect of guilt with which I'm all too well-acquainted... Capital "G" Guilt.

Every neurosurgeon who lives his/ her life on or near the edge of the serious-disease envelope has made at least one catastrophic mistake: if you haven't yet, you're on a short waiting list. These iatrogenic tragedies aren't common, but they're not rare either. The anatomical tolerances in the head and spinal canal are small, the brain and cord are fragile, and the consequences of even minor error are frequently disastrous and almost always irreversible. Those aren't excuses, just facts.

An error that costs a patient's life or health is the most horrible complication in a neurosurgeon's professional life; if possible, it's even more horrible the second time the error is made, even after a twenty-year interval. The ultimate in horror is when a student in his teacher's stead makes the mistake. No matter how many patients ultimately tell you they are alive and well because of your skill, experience or good fortune, it will always be those you've harmed in trying to save that will stay with you forever. The passage of time dulls that razor of agony to some degree, so if a guilty neurosurgeon can avoid self-injury or a career change in the first 48 hours or so following a fatal mistake, he or she probably has an opportunity to make a comeback. But the pain will never go away. There's nowhere to hide, no pill to take, no confessor to beg for absolution. I believe these mistakes are the best argument for the existence of hell, because they can never be reconciled in a single lifetime.

This type of ferocious, consuming guilt is a professional secret that only members of the club recognize.

It's rarely admitted and almost never discussed even among close colleagues. It has ruined promising careers and worse, has gutted some surgeons of the willingness to risk in order to cure. It leaves no life unchanged. As well as I can determine from both personal experience and close observation there's no reliable way to prepare for or even to anticipate the intensity of this emotion, nor to mitigate its impact. One simply has to live through it.

Chilling self-awareness of this type of personal guilt is by far the most intense emotion I've encountered in the practice of medicine, and just another small thing that went unmentioned in medical school. But, even in the setting of formal neurosurgical training, our emphasis as teachers is on errors and their prevention; there's little mention or focus on mitigation of surgeons' reaction to mistakes and their consequences. This is an important issue if fallible surgeons are to survive and grow, but currently, close observation and intrusive one-on-one mentorship are the sole recognized methods to limit the potential for damage.

In response to these powerful emotions of denial, anger and guilt, physicians (including this one) have developed an array of maladaptive responses to deal with the intense internal conflicts brought on by patients' morbidity and mortality. Not every surgeon is guilty of all- or indeed any- of these behaviors but they are in common usage in every practice environment I've experienced, and frequently physicians appear completely unaware of their use.

ESCAPE AND EVASION (A.K.A vanishing)

Despite what a layperson might imagine, there are several ways for a physician to limit his or her intimate contact with any specific in-patient or family member. Making rounds at odd hours, visiting with a large entourage in tow, signing out to a colleague or arranging for spontaneous weekends off; all these will provide the physician an amazing amount of free time and space for avoiding controversy, confrontation and failure while waiting for the world to turn, for this bad situation to resolve itself, for the disease to run its course. It's similar to hanging out within earshot but out of range at the OK Corral. The unpleasant truth known to us all is that you can't hide forever, and if, in a time when both patient and family have the greatest emotional need for your presence, you're completely unavailable, the basic contract between patient and physician has been completely breeched. The doctor's heartfelt wish to "just vanish" is a completely understandable aversion response; every physician understands its almost visceral allure. Unfortunately, to succumb to it is moral cowardice.

SPREADING THE BLAME

Another maladaptive approach to dealing with dying patients is especially popular in our large teaching hospitals. This diversion entails enlisting as many other professionals as is humanly possible in the patient's care. This is not heavy lifting because the list of potential consultants for a sick neurosurgery patient is limited only by the attending surgeon's imagination and / or the potential consultants' naiveté. This approach is especially easy for "uber" specialists like neurosurgeons, since realistically we don't know anything about any part of medicine distinct from the nervous system and everybody knows it. In addition, there are almost always multiple problematic issues involving other organ systems in these patients ripe for investigation. Unfortunately, this mode of distancing is greatly facilitated in environments where informal but definite "routine consultant" arrangements exist for essentially all neurosurgery patients.

'Spreading the blame' is easier now than previously, with the availability of neuro-critical care specialists in almost all in-patient neurosurgery venues. While these practitioners without question elevate the quality of care for neurosurgery patients, they not only diffuse blame for patients' ultimate outcomes but simultaneously provide a convenient surrogate / shield from family concerns that's difficult for the surgeon to decline.

FUTILE CARE

A final tactic, akin to both vanishing and spreading the blame, represents a major ethical and financial dilemma for American healthcare. If, when faced with a well-defined medically-hopeless situation, a physician wraps him or herself in the dirty shirt known as "doing everything possible," the surgeon not only diffuses responsibility but simultaneously insulates herself against any suggestions that she may have overlooked a therapeutic opportunity, or- God forbid- withdrawn care "prematurely".

This approach, often colloquially referred to as "covering your ass", squanders medical resources, raises unrealistic hope where none exists and needlessly protracts the agony of dying. In polite company, this process is referred to as "futile care."

"Futile Care" is a hot topic today in the sub-specialty areas of critical care medicine and Medical Ethics. Any real, in-depth discussion of this topic lies beyond my capabilities; however, it's a fact that in many cases of advanced brain injury or irreversible neurological deterioration, clinicians resort to "pulling out all the stops", not to benefit the patient who is beyond benefit, but to mitigate their own feelings of inadequacy, denial, and guilt. The futile care approach, unlike vanishing, is superficially very family- friendly, since naturally friends and family feel best when told "we're doing everything known to medicine," as opposed to hearing, "There's nothing we can do other than make her comfortable." With futile care everyone lives a lie, at least for a while, and we all ultimately pay for it.

Obviously, the maladaptive behaviors I've described above don't always occur in sequence nor do they appear in the face of every instance of patient morbidity /mortality. They do however rear their ugly heads frequently and sometimes repetitively in the professional lives of busy neurosurgeons. Not surprisingly they are reminiscent of behavior patterns previously identified and quantified in periods of great emotional and psychological stress. They have strong parallels with the five stages of grief initially described by Elizabeth Kubler-Ross, an insight which completely eluded me until I was grappling with a description of their presence in my own practice.

ACCEPTANCE

Before I came to that belated realization and began to review Dr. Kubler-Ross' work, my personal understanding of the importance of acceptance, the final stage described by Dr. Kubler-Ross, had been capsulized in a late-night telephone call with Dr. Charles Drake, the famous Canadian neurosurgeon Dr. Drake, my personal hero and sometime confessor, told me; "The very best surgeons admit, accept and endure. Somehow, they find the courage to risk again, but they never forget. And, they can never forget to share."

I don't believe Dr. Drake ever forgot a complication; more importantly he never forgot the patient who suffered the complication. But that last sentence- the importance of sharing- brought into focus his belief that these personal catastrophes had tremendous relevance to the emotional health and stability of other practicing neurosurgeons.

Acceptance itself is difficult to define; perhaps it's a little easier to get a handle on by thinking about what it's not. For instance, Kubler -Ross was adamant that while acceptance is often confused with the notion of being all right or OK about what happens, that's just not the case. Acceptance, in her view, is not about agreement; it's about reality testing, about cold-hearted analysis, and finally about moving forward while looking back. The morbidities and mortalities experienced by a neurosurgeon's patients inevitably change the surgeon's life and his relationship with his career. Acceptance for Kubler -Ross, and for Charles Drake, was to forgive but remember: to embrace the new reality, like it or not, and to craft the future around it.

For me, acceptance has been made a little easier by the realization I've tried to do the right thing, I've had more good days than bad, and that I've won some of these struggles. On the whole, I believe I've made a positive difference in patients' and families' lives. From time to time, it also helps a little to remember we weren't treating the measles.

CHAPTER TWELVE

Heal Thyself

A little, or in some cases a lot, of first-hand experience on the other end of the physician -patient equation should be a required course in medical school and / or residency training programs. There's no way to practically make that experience feasible, but it would be a sobering learning opportunity for would-be young doctors, a large majority of whom have never been sick or injured and many who have not previously been up close and personal with illness. Often as a physician or medical student, armored in a white coat and surrounded by your posse, you find yourself weaving your way with a somber look through a population of pain and suffering, all the while murmuring an esoteric, incomprehensible language in hushed tones. If you're not careful, the whole ritual can make you believe somehow, you're above it all. There's nothing like a breath of mortality to get you centered again.

During Spring Break of 2002, I took my two sons, Daniel aged 12 and Gabriel aged 10, to New Mexico for a ski trip. My wife, their mother Patricia, was spending three days at a medical meeting in Chicago and was planning to join us post haste. I'd been skiing episodically for several years and was a marginal intermediate while our sons were pretty accomplished beginners not far from catching up to old Dad. It hadn't been a great snow year in the southern Rockies., and the snow report the prior week had been "slushy". We were on the tail end of a hard freeze, so conditions had overnight turned to "icy", but hell, it was what we had, and we weren't going to do anything dangerous anyway.

Because of all our rudimentary skill levels, our family hadn't yet made any big investments in ski equipment, so the day prior to hitting the slopes we dropped into one of the local shops to rent the whole nine yards: skis, boots, and poles. Then I splurged, buying all three of us helmets, which were just beginning to appear on American slopes. Patricia, a trauma surgeon, is a self-confessed safety psycho- maniac and I'd seen two horrible skiing head injuries in adults, both of whom had hit trees while drunk, so we were both big believers in as much squash protection as one can buy. We also picked up some sexy looking amber snow goggles that I was pretty sure made me a dead ringer for Clint Eastwood, and in a drug store next door I bought two Cohiba cigars to smoke up on the mountain.

Early the next morning we were up and at them, or as much as you can be when the ski area is 17 uphill miles away on a very narrow two-lane road which didn't get plowed/sanded until about 10 in the morning. The views going up and coming down are truly majestic, but the state of New Mexico spends such a pittance on infrastructure that you're crazy to take your eyes off the pitted black top for more than a second. Despite the best efforts of some of the other nuts on the road we made it up to the parking area unscathed, unloaded our junk and trudged into the poured concrete "Main Lodge" which wasn't a lodge at all but rather kind of a big block house with a cafeteria, ski rental, ticket office, a "lounge" and an infirmary where all the Ski Patrol hung out.

We got lockers for our stuff before I went to the ticket office to sign up for a morning's worth of instruction for the three of us. In my limited experience, there's never much residual wisdom left over from the last ski trip a year ago, so a little instruction is a cheap investment to start off a safe trip. Chip was the name of our instructor, a local guy about fifty who seemed like a straight shooter so when he asked us about our level of competence I didn't gussy it up a bit. The kids were sorta like" Well, you know we're pretty good for our age, "but that old dog wasn't hunting with Chip. He said, "Yup, we'll start out with something pretty straight-forward." So, we loaded the lift without anybody getting dragged and took off uphill to Thunderbird, a run that the ski map described as "easy intermediate." Standing at the top of the run, "easy intermediate" wouldn't have been my exact description but like diving boards, the runs always look higher when you're looking down. Chip gave us some last-minute advice, said the run was slick and icy, so use the edges and cut good turns. Dan took off first like a pro and Gabe went chasing him, so before I moved they were both almost half way down the run. Pushing off, I squatted a little to cut my first turn, didn't get the edges in and went down like a big dog. I knew I was really going to bust my ass, but then my right binding didn't release, and the tail of my ski caught in the ice.

When the cartwheeling was over, I knew I was hurt pretty badly. Chip squatted down beside me and said he'd release my ski, so I could stand up, but I told him just to hold my boot when he released it from the binding because I'd broken my leg. He tried to tell me I was wrong, so I pulled rank, told him I knew what was what, that I had a fractured femur. I lay back on the ice, but when I wiggled my right leg just a little it felt like someone was tearing it off, so I bent the knee a tad and when the shock subsided, I heard Chip on his radio asking for help. Looking down slope I could see the two boys; Daniel was motionless, staring up at me, and poor Gabriel was trying to scramble back up hill in his ski boots. That's the only time I cried.

The Ski Patrol was all over us in just a couple of minutes, but every time a new guy arrived, he'd say: "Can't we get him up on his feet?" Finally, they came to the consensus opinion I might know what I was talking about, so when the sled arrived, the guy in charge asked, "Doc, can we lift you up without giving you anything?" I told him that just taking deep breaths was agony; without any more twenty questions he slipped my arm out of the ski jacket and gave me 8 mg of IV morphine sulfate. I could have kissed him as four guys gently lifted me, and my broken leg, out of the snow and on to the sled.

If you've skied much you've seen casualties coming down the hill on the Red Cross sled behind a couple of these Ski Patrollers. Just for your information, even with a good slug of morphine on board it's a pretty rough ride. Not only are you hurting, but also beginning to think about pitching what's left of breakfast to lighten the load. Fortunately, I made it down the short run to where the boys were waiting without throwing up, and then was busy calming them down for long enough that impulse went away. I wouldn't have minded vomiting because I knew with any luck I'd be going to the OR pretty quick but the jerky movement would have been more than my broken wheel could tolerate.

A big boxy ambulance van was waiting by the infirmary, and with me and the boys in the back and the two paramedics watching my vital signs we made it down the hill and to St Patrick's Regional Medical Center in about 35 minutes by my watch. I had a little history with St. Pat's; the previous year I'd been asked to do an external review on one of their neurosurgeons who had a lot of complaints from patients, physicians, nurses, you name it. Turned out he was absolutely terrible, and we ultimately got his license, but during the review I developed the strong impression that the hospital itself wasn't exactly first class. That said I was damn glad when we pulled under their portico.

The morphine was wearing off, so the ambulance to-ER transfer wasn't a walk in the park. That pain was nothing like the experience when the ER doc tried to take off my ski boot. I wouldn't have been surprised if my troops back in Dallas had heard that protest. Subsequently the doc was really sweet about postponing the ski boot removal until he could get an IV and another 8 mg. of morphine in me. Now we were talking; I don't remember having my clothes cut off or getting the x-rays taken or frankly very much for about the next thirty minutes.

Let's call the ER doc, who I loved dearly because of the morphine, Roger. At some point around here, Roger came prancing in with my films, turned the overheads around so I could look at them and then said, almost proudly, "You, Doctor, have a spiral fracture of your femur, and it's a doozy."

No shit, Roger. My thighbone was in three loosely connected pieces, the fracture line spiraling down from my hip almost to my knee. Even a brain surgeon could tell this was going to take some creative piecework to put back together, but my big worry right then was the kids.

Roger had the young women at the ER desk on the horn to our medical center back home, trying to get in touch with my partners, because I had no idea how to reach Patricia. One look at that x-ray had confirmed my suspicion I was going to be unconscious pretty soon for a protracted time period. There was no way I was going to leave Gabe and Dan alone in the OR waiting room while I was getting wired back into one piece. I knew only two people here in New Mexico. Mike French was a Stanford classmate currently eking out a living as a part time author- part time realtor; we'd played on a basketball team together during a seven-month stay in France. He'd gone on to grad school at Northwestern and then moved to New Mexico with his wife, Pat, who'd sold us our condo. Fortunately, they were both in town. Coming over immediately, they swept up the boys and took them out for lunch prior to bedding them down in their new home. One problem solved, at just about the time I met my would-be surgeon whom I'll call Brad.

Roger brought Brad in to introduce him to his next victim, and at first glance, the guy seemed pretty smooth. About 50, decent looking, great tan and very relaxed. We traded a few names that we both knew at UCLA where he trained and had been on staff off and on for a decade or so before his recent move to the Land of Enchantment. He took a cursory look at my leg and didn't seem to be too impressed. Not a bad thing- when you're lying there on the ER table about to have some guy you don't know whack on you, you really don't want him to look appalled at the prospect. I, the other hand, was pretty impressed, because my thigh was about twice normal size and rapidly taking on the hue of a giant eggplant, but I figured Brad probably knew his business. I damned sure wasn't going to fly back to Dallas to get it fixed..

About that time old Brad came back in after looking at the x-rays; he wasn't quite so laid back on this trip. He described the fracture as a bad one, said it would take some doing to fix it and that even with good luck I'd be off work for probably 4-6 months . The morphine was wearing off by now, so I told him I was anxious to get the show on the road if he felt comfortable doing the job. He introduced me to the anesthesiologist who'd just gotten to the hospital and then took off for the OR. I told Roger I could really use a little help here while they were getting me tee' d up, and he was a life saver with another smaller dose of IV morphine.

Things got blurry even before they turned out my lights. I remember the OR having that cold, astringent smell all clean ORs have- it reminded me in a good way of home. Like most of my own patients, the last thing I said or tried to say was to tell my wife I loved her, then I got hollow and empty and went a way for a while. For about four hours, as I learned later.

I missed waking up in the PACU, so the first thing I remember was being violently nauseated as I was moved into my hospital bed. That was just par for the course for me since I've pitched my cookies early and often after every whiff of anesthetic I've ever had. The good thing was that immediately or shortly thereafter the love of my life showed up. Seeing Patricia didn't actually make me feel any better, but I knew damn well then I was ultimately going to be OK. When the person who cares most about you- a former ICU nurse who became first a general surgeon and then a trauma/ critical care specialist- is at your bedside, your anxiety quotient begins to subside back to near-normal levels.

Brad showed up later that day -or maybe it was the next morning- bringing with him the final x rays that had been shot in the OR. He explained that the fracture was worse than he'd thought and that I had a bunch of muscle wedged in the fracture line that had prevented him from getting the fragments in direct contact with one another. However, he'd shoved a titanium rod down where the center of my femur should be, connected it to the bone fragments with screws below my hip and just above my knee and then wired the whole thing together. He said the construct" wasn't perfect", but that he hadn't wanted to flay my entire thigh open to clean the interposed muscle out because that would have made it a "bigger operation". He thought things would heal the way he'd left them.

I've talked to a lot of patients after I've operated on them, but not once have I said I did less surgery than they needed because it 'would have been a bigger operation." The patient doesn't give a damn how big the operation was because 1) it's over; 2) he was unconscious for the entire thing; and 3) he wants the best shot possible at getting well. So, both Patricia and I felt from this moment on that we might have a real problem.

That worry became a little more acute as the physical therapist came into the room for my first therapy session. When she gently picked up my leg the only way to explain the horrible sensation was as if from mid-thigh on south the leg was on backwards. As soon as she stopped moving my thigh the nauseating sensation went away, but it came right back as she lowered it on to the bed. I didn't puke but it was close.

X-rays the next morning showed all the fragments were where Rod had left them, which meant they were all in the same general vicinity. There were quarter inch gaps between the fragments, which I assumed were filled with shredded muscle, but in general it looked better than the pre-op version. More or less.

Brad said he was happy and that once my "blood level" settled down we could start talking about flying back to Dallas. Big fractures bleed a lot into the tissues around them; rough calculation suggested I had about 1500 cc (three units) of blood jam-packed into the muscles of my thigh. If my hemoglobin level went down very much more- as it probably would for a day or so- I was going to need to be transfused. This part of New Mexico sits about 7500 ft above sea level, so you need all the red cells possible to trap what little oxygen is in the air. I wasn't wild about getting blood, especially from a medical system I didn't know much about, and what I did know thus far hadn't inspired much confidence in either of us, so going home had a lot of attractions for a whole bunch of reasons. When my nurse of the day showed up with a big crystal necklace that featured a rock about the size of a tangerine and told me she was a real fan of 'crystal healing" I got even more interested in traveling.

We stayed in New Mexico until my fourth post-op day when I got a medevac flight out to Love Field. Actually I should say the medevac flight came to get me, carrying one of my partners, one of our neuro-anesthesiologists and a longtime friend who was incidentally the best neurologist in the Southwest. I could have kissed each and every one of them anywhere they wanted kissed. I left St. Patrick's with a fresh set of x-rays, my latest labs and a message from Brad, wishing me well. He didn't make it to the room in person that day. The flight was a piece of cake, and within four hours I was being admitted to our university hospital where I'd practiced for the five years since it opened.

A couple of my first visitors were two ugly orthopedists- Adam and Charley- guys that literally wrote the book on "Big Trauma Orthopedics"; pelvic fractures, crush injuries, and as it turned out, big spiral femur fractures. I'd known them both for a decade or so- one had operated on my mother- and we'd taken care of a lot of trauma patients together, so it was kind of like a reunion, all big smiles and bullshit, right up until they held my x-rays up to the light streaming through a window.

I figured I had a problem when they said they needed to go out to the nurses' station to "use the view box". What they really needed was to get their stories straight before dropping the bad news on their new patient. So, I was ready when they slunk back in to tell me Old L.A. Brad had underkilled my fracture by a fair amount, and they thought there was a pretty good chance it wasn't going to heal.

Patricia and I talked it over with Adam and Charley for a while; I suggested they just take me back and fix it right the next day, but neither thought that was the optimal thing, at least for the moment. The risk of infection if they re-opened and extended my incision would be pretty great, and with all the metal they planned to put in, an infection would really be a bad deal. In addition, I was going require a fair amount of blood and finally there was an outside chance the damn thing would actually heal, although if it did, they admitted my femur would be short and crooked. Just perfect.

So, over the next three months I learned a lot about several things. First and foremost, I grew to understand the hard work and constant frustration associated with rehabbing from a serious illness, something I'd asked thousands of patients to do over the past thirty years. Physically and emotionally challenging, the rehab itself was a piece of cake compared with the feeling of emptiness associated with the sudden absence of a job that had been the center of my life since I'd been 26 years old. Finally, all the downsides were magnified by the uncertainty of recovery: would I ever be able to walk straight, run a step or really play with my sons?

As I said, these were struggles not unique to me in any way, but I was observing them from a unusual viewpoint. Most of the time I could be objective, realizing that, assuming all went as planned, these issues would be time-limited. More ominously, from early days I had a hunch something wasn't right with the leg. As I transitioned from crutches to a cane and then to hesitantly walking on my own the generalized pain in my thigh came and went. What stayed was that freaky sensation of instability, of dislocation every time I'd ask the leg to change position. The simplest act, like getting in the driver's seat, would nauseate me for just a second, and then the nausea would subside and I'd be fine -until I needed to get out. Naturally I told Charley and Adam who studied my x-rays which showed I was" laying down good new bone" and said they couldn't demonstrate any evidence of instability, although I didn't want them to try too hard. They encouraged me to plow ahead, saying, as I'd said so many times to my own patients, "we'll just have to see."

After about ten weeks of this I went back to first seeing patients and then operating a light load of small cases. I was very careful, but every time I'd isolate my femur and move it, there would be a brief flash of horrible sensation down deep. I still struggle to describe the feeling – as if part of my leg was lagging behind and letting me know it was pretty tenuously connected to the rest. Nothing to do but keep on keeping on, so I did, gradually making the transition back into a full practice at 3 ½ months from the injury.

About this time, I got a new fellow, a fully trained Kuwaiti neurosurgeon who came to spend a year with us learning blood vessel surgery. Smart kid, hard working, really enthusiastic and unlike a lot of folks going into sub-specialty medicine, he like interacting with patients at every level and was a pleasure to have seeing new patients in the clinic. On about our third clinic day together I'd been sitting down watching him examine a lady when it came time for me to do a little hands-on medicine, so I got to my feet and suddenly there was a sharp metallic "snap". I felt as if I'd been shot right above my right knee and the fellow said, "Oh, Jesus God."

With his help, I sat back down, apologized to the frightened patient and asked her to return to the waiting room. Over the next ten minutes, the pain lessened but didn't disappear, so I arranged for one of my partners to take over the remaining patients, and got a pair of crutches. When I stood, the nauseating sensation was back to stay, so I hobbled over to see Charley and Adam.

The x-rays showed that one of the screws passing through my femur to secure the titanium rod had snapped while the other one at that level was badly bent. The study also confirmed that the fracture lines between two of the three bone fragments were widening, meaning the whole damn thing was coming apart. The screws had bent, then broken in response to the fragments' motion.

Charley and Adam were not optimistic. We set a date a couple of weeks in the future to reconstruct the reconstruction, then I went home to talk to Patricia and the kids. It was a setback for me and the whole family; I'd lost four months of healing time, working time, family time, but we were fortunate that I wasn't going to lose my leg, my job, our home, our marriage etc. just because some asshole hadn't been willing to give me his best shot on a Saturday afternoon. I know better than most that all surgical "mis- adventures" don't end in a do-over, so a second chance is just that, a second chance to get well.

In some ways I was relieved, because maybe now that gut-wrenching wiggle every time my leg moved would go away. And it did. When I emerged from anesthesia in July, the first thing I did was lift my femur off the bed. It hurt like hell, but that was because they'd sliced my entire leg open from hip to knee, taken all the old instrumentation out, put a bigger rod and more screws in and then wrapped the entire length of femur tightly in stainless steel cable. It hurt, but it was fixed, and I knew it in the Recovery Room.

There were a few additional hurdles, but I was back at work in two more months and by Thanksgiving I could even walk without a cane. Both legs were the same length and aside from setting off alarms at the airport every time I went through security there wasn't much I couldn't do- except ski. I quickly went back to operating and continued at full speed for another decade without another thought about my leg. Needless to say, Christmas was pretty good for Adam and Charley for years to come.

After the last surgery, at my request Charley called Brad in New Mexico to give him some follow-up. Charley told me it was a pretty short conversation; Brad was polite but that was about all- not very interested in what happened after I left St. Patrick's . During my convalescence I wrote him a letter, detailing the course of events and making clear that I too had been on the wrong side of clinical decisions that I wished now I could have had back. Finding out you did something wrong is one of the ways you learn in medicine like in everything else. I got no response, which any way you look at it is impolite. I heard later from my friend Mike French that the guy was having some very public marital problems. Tough shit. I've been on the wrong side of that as well, but it never caused me to cheat on taking care of a patient.

One of the very special things about surgery as a career is that- done right- it represents an unfettered opportunity to care about your fellow man, but only if you refuse to recognize limits in what you'll sacrifice to alleviate a person's pain and misery. Occasionally, no matter how good you are nor how hard you try, the pathology will simply kick your ass, but it can never be allowed to happen simply because you were unwilling to make the effort.

For me to honor that that commitment, it helps to have a clear, personalized picture of that individual misery in my head. That's my vision of Gabriel trying to climb back up that ski run, of Daniel crying silently in the long ambulance ride to St. Patrick's, of Patricia's face when Charley was showing us those images, and the memory of that special feeling when I'd move my leg. That vision has made me a better doc. I'd really like to share it with L.A. Brad.

CHAPTER THIRTEEN

Arrogance vs. Ignorance

There's not much that uniformly pisses off American physicians as does the issue of medical malpractice, which is interesting because most of us know almost nothing about any aspect of it except that we hate the very concept. As is true with a significant amount of other important stuff, my generation of doctors had no formal exposure to the legal aspects of medicine in medical school or specialty training, so everything we learned was word of mouth from other docs, a classic case of the blind leading the visually impaired. All that information could be boiled down to the following: "Doctors good and noble; lawyers bad and greedy; patients stupid and ungrateful." Philosophically pretty dubious but operationally effective, and definitely designed to keep any illumination from creeping in.

I'd been in practice for a little less than a decade when I got a call from an orthopedic friend in private practice. We'd been residents together and I knew him to be a good doctor and a solid citizen. He said he had a buddy he'd played baseball with in college who'd become a lawyer, just starting out in practice an adjacent community. The lawyer had shown a case to my friend, asking for his advice; the orthopod said he thought I should look at it. Orthopedists, as a group, are generally nice guys but not overly sharp. "So, let me get this straight, bone doctor; this guy is a plaintiff's attorney with a malpractice case against a neurosurgeon, and you think I ought to help him?"

"I think you ought to look at the case, that's all. Just tell him you agree to look, to review it, with no obligation to do anything else. He's a good guy, it's a bad case and he'll pay you $100 an hour to look it over. Don't tell me you're too busy becoming a big wheel to do that."

So I called the guy, whose name was Dale Kline. On the phone he sounded about 14 years old; he was so excited when I said I'd look at the thing I was sure he was going to have to change his pants. When he brought the records over to my office later in the week, Dale actually looked like a teenager – kind of preppy and clean cut- but a teenager who had been around the block a couple of times. He'd grown up in a small Texas town, played shortstop well enough to get a full ride to Baylor, where he'd been a starter his last two years. Told me he'd probably have made the majors except that he couldn't hit a major league fastball, curve or slider and couldn't throw very well from the hole. We'd played different sports but had a lot in common.

DK was trying to break into law practice as a solo attorney and thus far wasn't having much luck. He didn't want to do divorce law (which he described as the lowest of the low) so he'd hung around the courthouse enough to get some small time criminal cases but was living on a shoestring when a member of his local Baptist church had sent this family to his office. After listening to their story, even though he knew absolutely nothing about medicine, he'd told them he'd take the case. They were poor white folks, probably one half-step up from the trailer park, with no money so he'd convinced them to sign a contingency contract, meaning he footed all expenses and got 30% of any settlement. If you're Melvin Belli that's probably OK, but if you're six months out of law school with a wife and small child, it's a hard way to make a living.

I asked him to tell me a little about the problem, but to leave off the drama; just the facts, if you please. The victim was the family's 14-year-old daughter whom I'll call Sandy. This young girl was in fact a ballet prodigy. At considerable expense to her blue-collar family she'd been dancing since the age of seven and supposedly had become the most promising young dancer in the entire metropolitan area for the last decade- he had the newspaper articles to back that up- and until the past summer had been a strong candidate, if not a shoo-in, for a scholarship at Julliard in NYC. She was unquestionably that good. Then at the start of the summer, she began to have trouble with her legs; they just didn't do what she told them and over a period of several weeks she got to the point she could barely walk. The family was distraught, and the girl wasn't really articulate enough to make good sense out of what she was experiencing. Their family doc was an osteopathic general practitioner who couldn't figure things out either, so he got some routine x-rays of her legs, pelvis and spine which showed nothing. On a repeat examination, he thought she might have some differences in her lower extremity reflexes, but that didn't ring any bells for him, so he decided to send her to see the only osteopathic neurosurgeon in town.

Since forever there's been conflict between the 90% of American docs that are allopathically trained, meaning carry the M.D. degree, and the osteopathically -trained physicians whose formal designation is D.O. The degrees of difference in basic beliefs have varied over time, but it's fair to say that osteopathic training has traditionally focused much more on concepts of spinal malalignment as the source of most diseases while the concepts of allelopathy encompass a broader view of disease causation and treatment, and are broadly accepted as the basic foundations of modern medicine as we know it. In the latter decades of the twentieth century, osteopathic medical schools became much more aligned with traditional medical education; currently graduates from both disciplines are accepted in post-graduate specialty training at major medical institutions. There remain some isolated osteopathic specialty training programs which tend to be very small and located in very suspect hospitals; graduates of these institutions are rightfully looked on with real suspicion and have a hard time practicing anywhere other than in the isolated osteopathic community.

One of the initial environments that mixed and mingled D.O.s and M.D.s successfully was military medicine. I got my first experience with that situation during the thirteen months I spent as a staff neurosurgeon at Clark Air Force Base Hospital just at the end of the Vietnam War. Several of the docs on staff were osteopaths; they were routinely first-rate physicians. Right before the end of my tour, I came down with a vicious gastrointestinal infection called Salmonellosis and spent one solid week on IV fluids and big gun antibiotics being taken great care of by a young D.O. internist who was a real stud. So, my head's on pretty straight about D.O.s, two of whom we've graduated from our own neurosurgery training program.

Unfortunately, in the mid-1980s the osteopathic hospital in question was a hotbed of terrible medical care; if you were on staff there it was because you couldn't get privileges anywhere else. However, there was a patient community in town that swore by, rather than at, these physicians and Sandy's family were true believers, so off she went to see Dr. Gray, who was the only osteopathic neurosurgeon in the state. I'll say a little more about Dr. Gray later.

He examined Sandy in the presence of her mother and then told the both of them he was sure she had early onset multiple sclerosis and needed to be treated with steroids. When two weeks of that didn't work, he said maybe she had a ruptured disc in her spinal canal, so he admitted her to the hospital for a test called myelography. This examination requires a spinal puncture after which a sample of spinal fluid is removed and sent for analysis then a small amount of radio-opaque dye is injected to mix with the remaining spinal fluid; images are made as the dye is moved up through the spinal canal by manipulating the x-ray table. If there is a disc or something else pressing on the spinal cord the dye will be deformed in a certain pattern revealing the problem and its location.

Dr. G told Sandy's family that the test was normal, proving to him she was suffering from some type of hysterical neurosis that was producing her weakness. The day after the myelogram, he had submitted a consultation request to the Psychiatry department, but before the shrink could show up, Sandy lost control of her bladder. Almost simultaneously her mother finally lost confidence in Dr Gray and transferred her daughter to an actual hospital down the street.

There a real neurosurgeon named Ray White took a long look at her, repeated the myelogram and found a large benign tumor blocking her spinal canal two inches away from where Gray had stopped taking x-rays. Later the same day Dr. White took the kid to the OR and removed the entire tumor in about two hours. That was the good news; the bad news was that although Sandy regained control of her bladder and was able to walk, permanent weakness of her lower legs prevented her from ever dancing again.

Reading through these medical records and looking at the botched myelogram made me want to puke; here was an uneducated clown whose combination of ignorance and arrogance had almost made a complete paraplegic out of a young girl whose only sin had been to trust him. As I wrote my report, my concepts about malpractice began to change considerably.

Dale won a big settlement for Sandy from Gray's insurance company. After a very similar case two years later when Gray had blundered into the large abdominal veins on the front of the spinal canal while trying to remove what he thought was a ruptured disc from behind, Dale and I made a trip down to Austin to testify before the State Medical Board, after which the Board suspended Dr. Gray's license to practice.

In the thirty subsequent years I've participated in about 125 medical malpractice cases, 80% percent of the time for the physician defendants, 20% for the plaintiffs. I 've reviewed alleged malpractice cases for the US Government, the US Army, Navy and Airforce, the States of Texas, New Mexico, California, Louisiana, Florida and Hawaii, the Provincial Government of Ontario and more malpractice attorneys than I can name. In the same time frame I've personally had five malpractice suits filed against me, three of which were dropped; the remaining two were settled out of court. From start to stop, it's been an eye-opening experience that's taught me a lot about medicine, a little about law, and more about people and the society in which we live. A few examples:

In 2005 I was referred a fifty-year-old man who had been hospitalized at another local facility with a ruptured aneurysm; he sounded pretty sick, they couldn't fix it and we had room, so I took him. The patient's name was Clark Weather; he was a commercial truck driver who'd never paid much attention to his health, so he was a chronic smoker, hypertensive and badly in need of a good dentist. He was what we call a "screaming grade three sub-arachnoid hemorrhage". That translates as a patient who has had a serious bleed from an aneurysm usually located on the small artery at the base of the brain which connects the circulation of the two hemispheres. This region of the brain is intimately involved in emotion and its expression, so injuries (such as hemorrhages) there often produce severe mood alterations, one of the most common of which is violent, aggressive behavior. Clark had it in spades.

It's very difficult to take care of someone who's trying to hurt you, so generally nurses hate being assigned to one of these post-bleed patients, especially because the severity of their brain injury precludes the use of medication to make them more tractable. If a patient like this is sedated, they begin to retain CO_2, their intra-cranial pressure goes up, they may re-rupture their aneurysm, they become more obtunded, and you basically don't know what the hell is going on, so long story short, you just can't safely sedate these patients. Therefore, the nurses must rely on physical restraints, which is another sorry story.

There are now very strict rules which appropriately limit the nature of physical restraints which can be used in patients, as well as when and how they can be employed. Most commonly, very active patients who need restraints are placed in a restraint vest which encircles their chests and attaches to the bed frame; in addition, they are placed in padded cuff restraints, usually on both upper and lower extremities, which are also secured to the metal bed frame. Patients who are not somnolent hate restraints and struggle against them violently and almost continuously, but patients who are somnolent rarely need restraining at all. In a neurosurgery ICU, the nurses usually are trying to deal with an otherwise healthy individual with a brain injury that makes them violently aggressive, a patient that can't- for good medical reasons- be sedated. It's an impossible and thankless job.

The biggest risk to a patient with a ruptured aneurysm is re-rupture, which carries a mortality rate of over 50%, so almost uniformly we want to get these aneurysms secured as early after they're diagnosed as is humanly possible. In Clarks' case that was the afternoon of his admission, when he got a quick, straight-forward, uncomplicated operation, doing away with his aneurysm and eliminating as much of the blood from his hemorrhage as was safe to do. This blood, packed around the brain's blood vessels, can ultimately cause them to spasm, a condition which is difficult to treat and potentially lethal, so during surgery we typically vacuum away as much of the tenacious clot as possible. But the surgery itself does nothing to return the patient to a lucid state, so Clark came out of the OR just as he went in, screaming and fighting.

There's one big difference in the management of these patients post-op; following operation there's no longer a worry about them re-rupturing their aneurysm. So, at that time generally we rely more on medication than on restraints for control, but it's still a pretty fine line to chill them out without making them comatose, meaning you err on being conservative with the meds. It's a fine line, one we missed with Mr. Clark Weathers.

On his second post-op evening, Clark went bananas. He escaped from his wrist restraints, climbed over the elevated bedrail, ripped out both IVs and tore off all his monitor leads. He was trying to pull out his Foley catheter when three nurses got him under control, gave him a small amount of IV valium as a sedative and then wrestled him back into bed. The resident on call told me the next morning that it had been a huge mess; blood, IV fluid and urine everywhere, etc. Thankfully, the one thing Clark hadn't done was injure his head; when the resident inspected his wound, everything was where we'd left it and a stat CT scan showed the inside looked as good as the outside, so we felt that all of us had dodged a bullet.

The remainder of Mr. Weather's convalescence was much less exciting, and we were able to let him go home with his wife on his 10th postop day, which is actually a little early for this type problem. As is typical with hemorrhages like his, when I saw him back three weeks later in my clinic Clark remembered none of the details of his hospitalization. On his second post-op visit at six weeks, we OK'd him to return to work, and I never saw him again, although he had scheduled appointments at three and six months. Five years later Clark Weathers filed a mal-practice suit against me and the Medical Center, alleging malicious negligence and practice which was below the standard of care. In specific, the suit claimed that I had knowingly left a two-foot long catheter in his heart, thereby exposing him to all manner of death and disability.

When I sat down with the plaintiff's hospital record to try to reconstruct what had happened to him in the post-op period, it became obvious without much effort how things had gotten screwed up. Sick

ICU patients get a routine chest x-ray well before the day begins every morning; the films are reviewed by the neuro-ICU staff shortly after they're taken; however, the radiology staff, who dictates the formal readings doesn't do its work until late morning and the dictated reports don't hit the charts until early afternoon.

When Clark bailed out of bed in the middle of the night, he ripped his IVs out (one of which was a central line that extended from his forearm up to his heart); somehow, he severed that long intra- venous catheter leaving the segment in his upper arm and chest in place but dislodging the rest to drop in the mess on the floor. Error #1: no one inspected the remnants of the catheter to insure it was intact. Clark's chest film the following morning was unchanged from the previous day; he still had an indwelling central catheter, but the radiologists didn't know that it wasn't attached to an IV bottle on the other end, and the neuro-ICU team didn't look at the report the following day, a report which stated that the position of the catheter was unchanged. They're the only ones that knew the central line wasn't replaced after the midnight madness. Error #2; nobody connected the dots nor did any one order a chest x-ray after Lewis had left the unit.

When tort reform was passed in Texas in 2003, one of the new statues was mandatory mediation, meaning that both the plaintiff and the defendant, along with their attorneys, must meet together with a mediator to determine if some reasonable resolution of the claim can be reached before going to court. I think this is a good thing for both sides because it gives everybody a face-to-face opportunity to examine the issues, instead of doing it all through the proxy of attorneys who, believe it or not, have a vested interest in stoking the fires.

Prior to my mediation session, our insurance carrier's attorney, a smart woman of about 45, warned me that I was going to hear some accusations that wouldn't be pleasant, above and beyond the story of the IV catheter fragment. I shook that off as just boilerplate lawyer BS, but lo and behold, she was correct. Clark and his lovely wife had testified under oath not only had I personally and knowingly left the piece of catheter behind, but in addition, the last time I'd seen him in clinic I had said to them, and this is their quote," Mr. Weathers, I've made you better than God did."

Part one: I'm not an outwardly religious person. I have no formal church affiliation and Patricia is a lapsed Catholic; consequently, we raised our kids without consistent exposure to any particular faith. But I am a believer; you can't look at the marvel of the human brain every day for forty years without thinking there's something majestic and purposeful behind all our lives. That belief, if it does nothing else, makes a guy humble; I'm more than aware that the little I can do to make people healthy is insignificant in comparison to the power, the complexity and the majesty of creation. So, I'm pretty unlikely to compare my efforts to those of the creator, even if I'm not quite certain what to call him/her/it.

Part two: I have a visceral hatred for lies, for the people that tell them, and consequently, for the people that encourage the people that tell them.

So, by the time I process this specific piece of utter bullshit, I'm raging mad at these two conniving low- lifes and their equally conniving scum-bag of an attorney. Doctors don't go into surgery for applause; the privilege of doing the work itself is an incredible blessing. However, we damn sure don't expect to be vilified by the very folks we try to help, so my response to Clark, his lovely wife and their shit-head attorney was immediate, hostile and profane. Not much left to say, so that first mediation session wound down pretty quickly.

These mediations are set up to try to keep the conflict out of court; in a little piss-ant situation like ours, everybody knew going in that we were going to pay them some money and they were going to drop the suit. The question was, how much money and were there going to be any conditions for either party in dropping the suit. Even though it's the medical school's insurer's money, the accused physician has the final say about what happens; it couldn't be any other way, or you'd never get docs to agree to the insurance plan for starters. That said, any kind of trial costs big bucks even if you win.

It was going to be pretty much a slam dunk to prove that I personally did not shear that catheter off in old Clark Weathers, nor did I know it was there, nor was I just too damn lazy to take it out. But the fact was, we as a hospital system had allowed him to be discharged without recognizing or removing this catheter, and although he suffered no harm from its retention, he did have to undergo a thirty-minute catheter procedure to have it removed. So we were going pay, but probably not very much.

But we weren't going to pay a nickel in the presence of that bald-faced lie; I made certain our attorney knew it as soon as we left the conference room. I didn't give a rat's ass about Mr. and Mrs. Weathers "dropping the charges" because that was going to happen at some point regardless, but I wasn't going to bargain with that false allegation on the table. I'd been to court before and the prospect didn't scare me. And we were all going again, regardless of how much it cost, if the Weathers didn't get their shit together. So, I left them all to chew that over and went back to work.

Things worked out about as you might expect. After "due consideration" Mr. and Mrs. Weathers allowed as how they had perhaps "misheard or misinterpreted Dr. Samson" at the post-operative visit when I told the sorry son-of-a-bitch he was healthy enough to return to work. With that assertion removed from the formal charges, the Medical School's insurance plan paid the cost of his catheter removal and a grand total of $40,000. His dirt-bag attorney got thirty percent. When Clark filed for total and permanent disability six months later, he was denied. Shucks.

While the outcome of many of these cases turns on a subtle medical issue or a fine point of law, there are ones that pop up from time to time that are simply hideous mistakes which make it hard to believe that the accused clown ever got a medical license, much less escaped unscathed from a five-year neurosurgical training program. When these egregious errors occur, the guilty party is frequently somebody practicing by himself, having minimal contact with other neurosurgeons who might act as a restraining influence. Nobody is smart enough on his own to be right every time, but if you have to put your bright ideas into actual words and explain them to a colleague, most of the time the real stinkers get weeded out without anybody being hurt. If you're just talking to yourself, who knows what the hell you'll come up with?

This scenario cropped up in a case I reviewed for the defendant's attorneys relatively recently. As a general rule, I have tried to avoid passing judgement on a doc that I know personally for reasons related to potential conflicts of interest. However, in this specific instance I only knew of the guy, who practiced in another southwestern state, by reputation (which was poor) and I did know the attorney well, so I agreed to look at the case just to tell the lawyer exactly what kind of mess he had, rather than to be a so-called expert witness for his client. No money was changing hands.

This neurosurgeon- Dr. Blue- was notoriously lazy so it wasn't a big surprise on opening the chart to learn that the first issue related to the accused refusing to accept a patient in transfer from an out-lying hospital. Our hero was on call for the ER when he learned via telephone call that an elderly gentleman in a small town about forty miles away had suffered a stroke; according to the ER doc there, the patient needed to be transferred so that somebody could take out this huge clot in his brain that was probably going to kill him pretty quick otherwise. Most of what we call "strokes" are brain injuries that occur when the brain isn't getting enough blood supply, but 10-15% happen when a small blood vessel within the brain bursts, usually because of the long-term effects of uncontrolled hypertension. These "hemorrhagic strokes" are more lethal than the first type and in some isolated cases you can save a life by getting the mass of the clot out of there. That said, in most patients, emergency surgery doesn't help, especially if it's been a big bleed.

To our lazy neurosurgeon talking on the phone to the local ER doc, this situation sounded like the latter rather than the former, but he wasn't looking at either the patient or his CT scan. Nonetheless, he encouraged the local guy to admit the patient to his small hospital there and tell the family there was nothing that could be done to reverse the situation. The ER doc wasn't buying it; after they'd exchanged pleasantries, the patient was put in an ambulance and pointed toward the big city. The ER guy's transfer note reportedly ended, "Fuck you very much" although I didn't get to see the original.

To safely transfer the patient, whom I'll call Travis, it was necessary to provide him a secure airway, which meant the ER staff put a tube down through his mouth into his trachea, a procedure that requires a short-acting sedative given by IV push. This generally renders the patient unconscious and non- reactive for around four minutes, more than enough time to get the tube in, safely secured to the face and then attached to a ventilator. The only situation in which the effects of the medication may be prolonged are if the patient is an alcoholic with advanced liver disease, because the sedative is metabolized exclusively by the liver. Everybody knew Travis was a lifelong drunk, his ER chart even said so.

Well, when Travis hit the big city ER, the emergency room staff got him bedded down, ordered a new CT scan (because additional bleeding is pretty common) and then paged Dr. Blue, who showed up about the time the scan was completed. There was, in fact, a little increase in the size of the clot but it had already been big enough to be fatal, so if it was going to be removed, that had to be done right now. Blue scanned the transfer notes, looked at Travis cursorily (his written physical examination is an embarrassment) and then went out to tell the anxious family that unfortunately Travis had died. He explained about the clot, said it wouldn't have mattered if the bleed had happened right here in town because nothing could have been done as the hemorrhage had destroyed the critical brain centers that control respiration and heartbeat. He commiserated with them briefly, then left for his office, after writing a brief note in the chart declaring the patient met the clinical criteria for brain death.

When the family went in to pay their respects, Travis was trying to sit up on the examining table. Paralyzed on one side, his good arm had just jerked the endotracheal tube out, which set off the ventilator alarm, resulting in a Code Blue resuscitation protocol, which is something a family should never witness. People come swarming in from all over the hospital with their hair on fire; in seconds nurses and doctors are pounding on the patient's chest, jamming another tube down his throat, yelling at one another and just generally creating chaos. When the smoke cleared, it was obvious that although he was really sick, Travis was still alive and kicking.

I would love to hear a recording of the ER physician's subsequent telephone conversation with Dr. Blue, but unfortunately none exists. The ER chart notes themselves are very cryptic; they explain that this patient who had been previously declared dead apparently had a respiratory arrest after extubating himself. A "full code" was successful in re-establishing an appropriate airway and Travis was undergoing "re-evaluation" by the neurosurgical consultant. No kidding.

Dr. Blue maintained that the patient had indeed been brain dead (the first of the brain death criteria states that the patient cannot have received any paralytic or sedative drug in the past eight hours) and that in fact if he had gotten such drugs, they would have worn off in the hour plus transit time between hospitals, regardless of Travis' liver disease. "This is inexplicable," he wrote, but now that he had a live patient, he was willing to take Travis to the OR for clot removal. The family didn't have much choice, but when Travis did finally die two days after surgery, they were less than happy with Dr. Blue's care.

Within a month, they'd filed suit, alleging Dr. Blue's inability to diagnose death had been below the standard of care expected of a neurosurgeon in this particular state.

Malpractice law is unique in that there are two parts to convicting a practitioner. The first is that the jury must agree that whatever the doc did, or didn't do, was substantially different than what any other reasonable physician with the same background and training would have done, possessed with the same information in the same or a similar situation. Part two is that the jury must be convinced that, more likely than not, the physician's aberrant behavior resulted directly in harm to the patient.

I told my attorney buddy that while part one was a slam dunk in Travis' case, proving that the delay associated initially with Dr. Blue's refusal to accept the transfer and then ultimately in his missed diagnosis negatively affected the ultimate clinical outcome was going to be a much harder lift. Over 90% of patients with hemorrhages the size of Travis' will die as result of the bleed regardless of whether or when their clot is removed; when you factor in his terrible liver disease and long-standing hypertension, Travis' chances for survival were miniscule from the get-go.

I suggested it would probably be easier to convince a dozen neurosurgeons of that, rather than a jury of twelve folks from the community, and the attorney agreed. The case was ultimately settled out of court for something like $250,000, and Dr. Blue went under the scrutiny of the State Medical Board, who apparently thought being able to identify a dead patient was an important neurosurgical skill.

Surgery of spinal disorders has long been a subspecialty claimed by both orthopedic and neurosurgery, a competition that was pretty benign until the mid-1990s when simultaneous developments in imaging and implant technology made it at least theoretically possible to correct any bony spinal anomaly as long as the surgeon was willing to do a big enough operative procedure. In many ways this proved to be a boon to patients who suffered from crippling spine related- diseases or traumatic spine injuries, but symptoms aren't always directly related to x-ray findings and one of the loosest correlations is between back pain and "disc disease." The intervertebral discs, located between vertebral bodies, are composed of a thick fibrous ring (the annulus) which connects the bones and encloses a gooey, cartilaginous substance called the nucelous pulposas. This latter stuff has a high water content and ideally serves as the spine's shock absorber; it's flexible, compressible and spares the bony components of the spine much of the repetitive trauma of flexion and extension.

Unfortunately, like all the body's parts, the two components of the intervertebral disc are subject to the dual ravages of injury and aging. Both the annulus and the nucleus lose part of their water content as the body ages: this means that the annulus becomes more brittle and the nucleus shrinks, allowing more motion at the disc space, and permitting the cartilaginous component to fragment under stress. So, the infamous "ruptured disc" is most commonly a situation induced by repetitive trauma which produces a tear in the brittle annulus followed by an extrusion of portions of the nucleus. That all sounds pretty benign but because of the way the spine is assembled, this extrusion comes to lie in the narrow spinal canal where it exerts pressure on the spinal cord or, more often, the nerve roots leaving the cord and exiting the canal to form the major nerves that serve the arms and legs. The cord and the nerves themselves aren't pain sensitive, but the membrane covering both (the dura mater) is exquisitely pain sensitive to the pressure from these "herniations". Trust me; I've had a couple.

So, what with bony overgrowth, joint arthritis, excess motion, and disc rupture there are a lot of potential components to spine-related pain; almost always more than one is at play in any given patient. And there's no magic bullet that cures them all. So, the good spine surgeon has to be very particular in selecting his targets and even more careful in selecting his patients, if we assume his actual goal is to make the patient, rather than the patient's x-ray, better. Unfortunately, that's not always a valid assumption.

The changes in imaging and implant technology have, over the past two decades, spawned a geometric increase in the amount of spine surgery being done in this country... and some of it is indicated. Another contributor to the dramatic increase in spine surgery volumes is the enthusiasm with which hospitals have embraced it, and that is based solely on its lucrative financial benefits. Spine surgery has replaced heart surgery as hospitals' biggest money maker; when each one of six to eight screws used in a procedure costs $40 to manufacture in Japan and the hospital's charge to the patient's insurer is $400 (times six to eight), plus two rods at $800 apiece, four connectors at $500 each and two cross-links ($250 a pop) pretty soon we're talking real money . Add in the costs of intra-operative imaging, bone implants and assorted add-ons, and you're looking at the root of all evil.

Although surgical procedures to remove "ruptured discs" are among the most common operations in this country, they are far from being the simplest. Intervertebral discs are situated between the bony vertebral bodies in front of the spinal canal, but the easiest way to approach them surgically is via an incision in the midline of the low back. This incision is deepened to separate the large muscles of the lumbar spine, again in the midline, thus exposing the shingled, bony roof of the spinal canal known collectively as the laminae. One or two of these laminae must be removed to expose the interior of the canal and the dural tube enclosing the end of the spinal cord and the nerve roots that stream down from it. That tube must be mobilized, moved gently away from the lateral or side walls of the canal to expose the back, or posterior, wall of the disc and any herniated fragments pushing in under the nerve roots.

The standard operative procedure, once these fragments have been removed, is to gingerly open the back fibrous wall of the disc and then carefully explore the interior of the disc for any other free or degenerated components. This exploration involves blindly probing through tissue the consistency of cartilage, removing any portion thought to be abnormal with a slender grabbing instrument initially developed to remove pituitary tumors. Because the body's largest artery and vein lay tightly applied to the front wall of the disc and because this exploration is truly blind, this is the most dangerous portion of the operation, made even more risky because if one of these vessels is injured, there is no way to repair it through this incision. In the case of an injury, the patient must be hurriedly turned on to his /her back and an abdominal incision made to gain access to these huge arteries and veins, which meanwhile are pouring blood out through the site of injury. This is how patients die during disc surgery.

In 2010, I was asked to review a mal-practice claim on behalf of a defense attorney whose client, a well- known orthopedic spine surgeon, had the reputation of being a nice guy but a terrible surgical technician. In view of that reputation, I advised the attorney that I'd be willing to look at the records to determine what actually happened to the patient, but that I wasn't interested in being a witness for the defense. We went back and forth a little but ultimately, he agreed on a price and sent me the records, which were extensive and incredibly obtuse.

The patient had indeed undergone lumbar disc surgery and had developed extensive bleeding intra-operatively requiring the emergency intervention of a vascular surgery team to repair not one but two lacerations of the huge vein in front of the spinal column. The story didn't end there unfortunately, because in the post-op period the patient had developed a serious intra-abdominal infection that necessitated re-exploration and protracted intra-venous antibiotic administration. After almost two months hospitalization, much of it in intensive care, he'd been discharged to a chronic care facility, essentially disabled by both his back pain and his abdominal wound.

The first time through the chart I thought this saga was a pretty straight forward, regrettable example of a vascular injury secondary to a "surgical misadventure" during lumbar disc surgery. Many spine surgeons unfortunately have one of these on their records. Even though the risks of a vascular injury are clearly stated in the operative consent form, that's not a vaccination against a malpractice charge, so typically, a significant amount of money changes hands and the thing is settled out of court without further ado. The hooker here was the post-op infection, not a common thing after a vascular procedure, but I really couldn't identify anything else. I called the attorney to tell him things looked pretty bad, although I didn't know whether legally this complication constituted mal-practice; maybe there was some theoretical protection because this was a recognized potential complication of the operation and the patient had signed the operative consent form.

He was quiet for a few seconds, then said, "What about the frozen section?"

It's never good when you're the "expert" and the lawyer knows more about the medical aspects of the case than you do. I swallowed a big chunk of crow and said I'd call him back.

Sure enough, the OR Nurses' notes contained the notation that Pathology had been summoned to the OR about ten minutes before the shit hit the fan to perform a frozen section analysis of a 'tubular" piece of tissue removed from the disc space by the spine surgeon. Before the subsequent pathology report could be returned, the vascular injury had been recognized and the remainder of the nurses' documentation dealt with efforts to compensate for the torrential hemorrhage, the hurried closure of the back incision, the patient being flipped into the supine position and the emergency laparotomy and vascular procedure which followed. But buried in the hundreds of pages of laboratory results was a single page pathology frozen section report which consisted of one phrase: "Specimen consistent with appendix." As far as I'm aware, it's the only appendectomy in recorded medical history to be done by a surgeon from the back by first making a large hole in the spinal canal and inferior vena cava. Hard to put much lipstick on this little pig.

One of the most regrettable causes of surgical error is arrogance, usually expressed something like this: " I've done 10,000 of these operations: the chances I'm going to fuck this next one up are less than zero." Any operation a surgeon undertakes without the haunting awareness in the back of his/her head that things can go to hell in a heartbeat should be referred to someone who routinely goes into the OR expecting disaster.

Perhaps the most classic two examples of this master-of-disaster mindset I encountered in my practice were the province of an overbearing, narcissistic plastic surgeon I'll call Dr. Cortes, and the first involved a 15 year old boy named Kevin. This young man had been born with a cleft lip / palate combination which had been skillfully repaired by Dr. Cortes at an early age. Post-op Kevin's appearance may not have been movie-star quality but there was damn sure nothing wrong with his brain. As a sophomore in high school his IQ was off the chart and he was blitzing through college level calculus and physics; the young man was almost guaranteed to be a lock for a full academic ride at a prestigious university.

At a routine follow-up visit with Cortes, Kevin and his parents wondered if something might be done to make his lip scar less obvious. The surgeon agreed that would be possible and added that while he was at it, he could easily correct Kevin's small degree of nasal septal deviation without breaking a sweat.

So, in the following summer, prior to Kevin's junior year, he was admitted for "scar revision and rhinoplasty".

The surgical procedure was unremarkable, but the fact that Kevin didn't emerge promptly from anesthesia was not. Even worse, twenty-four hours later when he did gradually begin to regain consciousness, it was apparent to everyone that something was badly wrong. He was stuporus, confused and intermittently aphasic. About the only communication his parents could decipher was that his head hurt horribly.

Dr. Cortes suggested this symptom complex might be some type of "conversion reaction", a mental state related to hysteria, but the consulting neurologist wasn't impressed with that diagnosis. Instead, he ordered a CT scan which showed the boy had suffered a large hemorrhage that essentially filled all the spaces around his brain. This type bleed is most often seen with a ruptured aneurysm, and on close examination of the ensuing arteriogram, a small, very unusual aneurysm was identified on one of the brain's major arteries in the midline, just above the roof of Kevin's orbits. Aneurysms in kids are infrequent if not exactly rare; however, aneurysms at this location on this specific artery are almost unheard of, unless they are related to penetrating trauma. Regardless of their origin, ruptured aneurysms, especially in children, must be surgically obliterated post haste, because the frequency of re-hemorrhage is very high and the mortality rate is greater than 80%. So, we took Kevin in transfer and shipped him almost straight to the OR.

The aneurysm was easy to find and gratifyingly simple to fix; it had been caused by a tear in the artery overlaying a discrete puncture wound in the skull base . The penetrating object had punched through the thin bone between Kevin's orbits, leaving a small flap of bone that looked through the microscope like a tiny trap door through which some bloody mucosa from the underlying ethmoid sinus protruded. After repairing the injured artery, we coagulated and then amputated the small tongue of bruised mucosa, patching the bony defect with a plug of methyl methacrylate, and taking photographs to document every step. Once we were closed, Kevin went back to the angio suite to prove the aneurysm was gone and the artery still intact. They were, so then I went out to the waiting room to talk to Kevin's parents.

After reassuring them their son was OK, I did a little preliminary ground work and then showed them the series of photographs of the injured artery, its repair, the trap-door-like defect with its tiny attached bony flap and finally the reconstituted skull base. Then came the hard part- their questions.

Both of these folks were intelligent and engaged; their questions were exactly what you would imagine and I answered them as frankly and completely as possible.

Two days later I got an irate phone call from Dr. Cortes. I told him what we'd found and done and then listened to him regale me with the many thousands of rhinoplasties he'd done with nary a complication one. Well, I said he had one now. After listening to a little more bullshit, I faxed him copies of all of the intra-op photos, complete with labels in case the anatomy was unfamiliar. I asked him to call me back with another explanation when he came up with one, but added that for the moment, we were going to ride with the truth.

From a neurosurgical viewpoint (which often is a pretty low bar) Kevin made an adequate recovery; after a prolonged period of rehabilitation he regained most of his basic motor and communication skills and could pass for normal if you didn't look too hard. Unfortunately, much as was true with my friend Dr. John Shepherd, his ability to reason, to remember and to think deductively was permanently lost. The subsequent malpractice suit was settled out of court before my scheduled deposition was taken.

Arrogance, at least in surgeons, seems to be a pretty durable trait, refractory to impact by negative experiences. I next encountered Dr

Cortes a couple of years later when I answered an unusual emergency page from the operating room of our adjacent Children's Hospital. From the get-go in 1977, I had limited my practice to adults, although I occasionally went over to Children's to consult on a child with a vascular problem. By this time there were two competent pediatric neurosurgeons on the Children's staff, and frankly I'd decided early on that the heartache of dealing with sick kids (and the headaches of dealing with their parents) simply wasn't a bonus I needed in my practice. So, this STAT page was truly strange, and when the OR operator put me through to Room 8, I had no clue.

The surgeon who came quickly on the intercom identified himself as a plastic surgery fellow; he hurriedly explained that a four-year-old girl was bleeding uncontrollably from a surgical wound in her head and would I please come help? Before starting my 200-yard dash, I asked him if there were any adults in the room. Sure enough, the girl was a patient of my old friend Dr. Cortes; in addition a young neurosurgeon who'd just come to town was also present and scrubbed.

As I hustled down the long corridor connecting the two hospitals, I racked my brain to figure out what these knuckleheads could be doing that could exsanguinate a four-year-old child. It couldn't be trauma- if the kid had a gunshot wound or something similar she'd be in the OR behind me at Metropolitan, being cared for by my troops and the Trauma team. I came up empty of answers, but once I was guided through the OR doors things immediately became clear. As in, crystal.

Kids tolerate massive blood loss very poorly, so you almost never walk into a pediatric OR that smells like a butcher shop, but this one did. Framed by the large semi-circular craniotomy, the blood streaming from a long laceration in the dura had the thin brown tinge of dilute grape juice; obviously anesthesia was far behind in transfusions and what little blood was there wasn't carrying much oxygen. Even worse, the rude mouth of the dural wound seemed to actually suck with each aspiration. Diagnosis wasn't a problem; the only thing that acts like that is a hole in the sagittal sinus, the brain's largest vein. Clustered around the child's head were two plastic surgery fellows (Plastics #1 and #2) and the young neurosurgeon whom I'd met socially. Sulking in the corner was good old Dr. Cortes, who didn't even have the balls to meet my eyes.

This was another re-operation gone bad. The child had been born with premature closure of one of the skull's sutures, the bony seams that normally stay open to accommodate brain growth during the first two years of life. Dr. Cortes had done a straight-forward operation at the age of six months to open that prematurely-fused suture and now was back to make the result more cosmetically acceptable. All well and good, except as the team had cut the bony flap and attempted to elevate it from the underlying dura, they'd managed to put this gaping hole in the sagittal sinus and now had no idea how to close it. Because of the pressure differential between the atmosphere and the interior of the vein, every time the surgery team raised the child's head to diminish the bleeding, the torn sinus would "suck" air and shoot it straight to the right heart, which wasn't at all amused. But when they lowered the head, the sinus bled like gangbusters . The combination of alternating air embolus and massive blood loss was about to kill the patient, who'd just come in for a little cosmetic "re-shaping."

For a neurosurgeon to accidently put a hole in the sagittal sinus is not a mortal sin, but repairing such a laceration is an essential skill; however there would hopefully be time for sorting that out later. I told Plastics #1 &#2 to put gentle pressure on the laceration while keeping the wound flooded with saline, then I made the neurosurgeon open the dura with a knife and a pair of scissors well away from the sucking wound. Once he had a decent hole I told him convert it into a large horseshoe-shaped incision with the open end of the horseshoe pointed at the laceration. Then I convinced him to elevate the dural flap formed by the incision from the underlying brain and reflect it down over the sinus laceration, once the plastic guys quickly removed their fingers. Just laying the thin sheet of dura down on the hole reduced the bleeding; negative pressure inside the sinus gently sucked the dura down into the laceration with respiration. As the bleeding slowed dramatically, I knew we had a winner if the kid was still alive. Unnecessarily as an afterthought I coached the neurosurgeon where to put his stitches as he tacked the flap down permanently.

Just about then the anesthesiologist let us know she had managed to transfuse enough blood to stabilize the girl's vital signs. She had no idea what had happened, but in a quivering voice said, "Thank God you all got the bleeding stopped!"

The three guys scrubbed shuffled around for ten seconds like they'd been caught with their zippers down, then the neurosurgeon looked up at me. "Thank you very much for coming- we might have lost her."

Thinking, "Might have?" I tapped him on the shoulder. "Buddy, it could happen to anybody, you would have figured it out...yadda, yadda."

I looked over at Cortes, but I guess the cat still had his tongue, so I headed for the door. Late that afternoon, I got a call from Plastics #1, who just wanted to say thanks again.

The following week I was seeing patients in my clinic when my long-time friend and nurse Linda told me there was an unscheduled person in the waiting room demanding to see me.

"Duke, she's out there crying her eyes out. I think you should see her."

Long story short, naturally our unscheduled visitor was the girl's mother. Although Dr. Cortes had told her that "we had some unexpected bleeding because of all the scar tissue, but no big thing- we got it stopped", she had heard a different version from the anesthesiologist and ultimately from Plastics #1, who also went out of his way to mention they'd had some help from over in the medical school.

Mom had run with that and found her way to my clinic just to say "Thanks." We were all pretty teary by the time Linda ushered her out the door. Surprisingly I never got a follow-up call from Dr. Cortes.

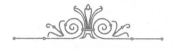

CHAPTER FOURTEEN

Wrong (Site-Side-Diagnosis)

Y ou'd think it would be pretty hard to operate on the wrong arm or leg. I mean honestly, one is broken or bleeding or swollen or something and the other one isn't; that's why the damn patient came to see you in the first place, right? You just look at the patient, check the x-ray and then get after it. Same deal with the ears, maybe not so easy with the eyes, especially if the problem is way back in there; that's an organ system to be very careful with, especially if the patient can't tell you which eye doesn't work. What about the head- by that I mean the brain?

Assuming the patient doesn't have a gunshot wound or a hatchet embedded in his skull, one side looks pretty much like the other, as in identical. Add to that the fact that if there's something wrong with one part of the brain it's usually the patient's opposite side that will be affected, but not always, and sometimes both sides won't be working all that well, plus other times everything is working because you're trying to prevent a tragedy, not reverse one. So not so simple.

Ah, you say-but what about the x-rays (or images as we call them now)? They always tell the truth and point the surgeon right at the badness, no? Well, like the images themselves, that's open to varied interpretation. Almost all the imaging used now to look at the brain and the spinal cord is computer- based; that is to say, CT scans and MR scans are images that are derived from computer-based receptors and are subsequently displayed on flat two-dimensional frameworks. The fashions and sequences of that display are totally arbitrary, meaning they've been selected from other equally valid candidates to be the single "right" way to look at the information. Who did the selection? Well, back in the early 70s, when CT was just coming on the scene, a bunch of radiologists (x-ray doctors) decided that the rationale for looking at a barium enema or a pelvic x-ray should apply to this new technology as well, regardless of what it meant for the doctors who were using the images to actually take care of people.

So, these clowns pushed through the idea that these new images should always be displayed as if the viewer were standing at the patient's feet, meaning that what's on the right side of the image you see is actually on the left side of the patient's head, and vice-versa. Despite a fair amount of protest from the troops in the trenches this viewpoint carried the day and going forward all CT and MR images of the brain and spinal column have been displayed in reverse orientation to the way an observer standing at the patient's head actually sees the real organs.

If you think this hasn't caused a few problems, imagine that every map or GPS display you looked at was portrayed as if you were viewing it from underground. That each image has a small font R to identify the right side hasn't prevented such problems is an established fact, and the whole controversy is just a classical example of what happens when non-clinicians have the ability to make practical decisions that will affect patients' lives.

Timothy, a ten-year-old boy, was sent to see me because he'd had a seizure; during its work-up, which included both CT and MR, he was found to have a nasty looking cavernous angioma located on the inside tip of his left temporal lobe. The referring doc didn't want to deal with the hassle of taking the thing out and as we talked on the phone, he mentioned that the other hassle he wasn't fond of was the boy's mother, who he described as a certified witch. I'm not sure which he liked less, Momma or the group of leather-clad bikers that stomped around with her and her son everywhere they went. I was never certain about the relationships there, but you can bet none of them involved soap.

Seeing Tim in the office I came to the conclusion that the cavernoma was going to be a lot less trouble than this mother who was completely obnoxious to everyone, not excepting me. She and her son had crappy insurance, so it took a major effort on the part of our billing folks and in turn the hospital's financial office to just get the kid cleared for admission and surgery. Instead of being grateful we were working our collective ass off to offer her son the best care possible, she was a giant pain in the butt to everyone she encountered. My nurse, one of the nicest people in the world, told me she was pretty sure Tim's referring doctor had spelled "witch' incorrectly.

We finally got all the hurdles jumped and Tim's surgery was scheduled for the following Wednesday, the only day of the week on which the ORs start at 0800, rather than an hour earlier. Everybody uses this extra hour to have a conference; for us in Neurosurgery it was Vascular Conference Day. We reviewed the images and case histories of the patients in-house and those we were seeing as out-patients, made treatment plans and tortured the residents about what little they knew about vascular neurosurgery. Our chief resident at that moment was an absolutely spectacular fellow I'll call Arnie, who ran the conference like a benevolent drill sergeant and made it a learning experience for everyone, staff and residents alike.

On the day of Tim's operation, the conference was running a little late. At 7:55 we still had one important patient to discuss. Arnie knew this last patient like the back of his hand, so rather than Arnie going upstairs to oversee putting Tim to sleep, I asked him to hang tight for the presentation, grabbed the image folder and headed up to Room Four.

The team wasn't waiting on us. Tim was asleep and ready to be positioned, which is one of the most important parts of a neurosurgical operation. Because all cranial operations are done through a small bony window in the skull, if the head is not in a position which takes advantage of the effects of gravity on the soft brain, making it move within the skull, an easy operation can be made very difficult and a difficult one a nightmare. During my practice, I always positioned the patients myself; if one of my assistants had jumped the gun, positioned the patient and put the drapes on, we just took them off and went back to square one. So, I hurriedly put the images up on the view box and then put Tim's head in a clamp-like set of tongs which would immobilize it during the operation. Looking over my shoulder at the view box, I turned his head almost into the lateral position, the way it would be if he were lying on his side on the OR table, and then tightened the clamps to secure it there.

The temporal lobe is situated just beneath the portion of the skull that lies immediately in front of and above the ear. It's about six inches long, three inches tall and extends down into the head about three inches deep. Tim's problem was located on the deepest surface of the front or tip of the lobe, probably four inches below the inside of the skull. I had a hunch I could get there through a small bony window about two inches by two inches placed right in front of his ear, an exposure which would let me use a straight skin incision beginning in his sideburn and rising up above the ear to be hidden behind his hair line. Always nice to spare the patient a visible scar if possible, but you can't cheat on the money part of the surgery worrying about the cosmetics; hell, then you'd be a plastic surgeon.

Arnie was still busy downstairs when I got Tim all prepped and draped. I'd used a small hair clipper to cut an inch-wide strip where I was going to make the incision, but the rest of his hair was intact. I figured Mom would at least love that. I injected the skin with our routine potion of lidocaine and epinephrine, which numbs sensation and simultaneously causes the skin's blood vessels to constrict, minimizing blood loss. After making the skin incision, I used the back of the scalpel to elevate the skin from the underlying muscle, so we could apply some clips that would prevent any bleeding later when the epinephrine wore off. I was just closing the last clip when Arnie came in.

He walked over to the view box, spent about thirty seconds there rattling the films around and then came up behind me as I was slipping a retractor in the wound to broadly expose the muscle. Next step was to open the muscle in a fanlike incision and scrape it off the skull, so we could get down to business. Looking over my shoulder, Arnie said, "Boss, where's the kid's nose?"

That's a weird question, but I figured he wanted to know how much I had the head turned. I put my hand down on the drape over the kid's face and answered," Right here."

It was real quiet for about ten seconds and then he said, "Boss, I think you're on the wrong side."

Everyone has probably experienced at least one episode of sudden terrible shock. Personally, the best I can describe the sensation is having a high volume, high pressure ice water enema but obviously that doesn't come close to doing it justice. At that special moment if your heart doesn't stop, and you don't puke or lose bowel and bladder control, you've probably got a chance to recover but you'll damn sure never forget.

I gave the knife back to Theresa our scrub nurse and then walked through a very silent OR over to the view box, where Arnie had left one film as I'd originally put it up, to show me I had had the sides reversed. No shit. I was on the wrong side of Tim's head and had a six-inch incision through the skin and down to the muscle to prove it. I shook my head, asked Arnie to scrub and told him how I wanted this ridiculous fucking incision closed. When he came back and gloved up, I stripped off my stuff and went out to walk around the OR suite for a while.

Bad mistake, can't make that incision go away but thank god I got stopped before getting any deeper. So, what now- go tell his crazy mother and her biker buddies that I screwed the pooch and wanted a do- over next Wednesday? The technical aspect of taking this thing out, even from the correct side, wasn't going to be exactly a slam dunk. Having made the incision on the wrong fucking side of the head, could I now settle down enough to do the operation the kid needed or was I going to be a bigger risk to Tim than the damn cavernoma? Could I stop thinking about how incredibly stupid I was and suck it up to do the right thing?

Well, this is what is known as a gut check- I'd already failed the brains check. Once we put a dressing on the incision, re-positioned Tim's head and got back to business, I had everyone's attention, and we were focused. The exposure was difficult enough to make me a little angry, which has always been really theraputic so by the time I got us down to the action we were smoking hot, and with about three strokes of the micro-knife, the damn thing just fell out. Elapsed time from scope to removal about twenty minutes. Total blood loss was about twenty cc's; back when I was still shaving with a straight razor I'd cut myself worse many a time.

With the cavernoma laying on the Mayo stand, I asked Arnie to remove the slick ring of stained brain that enclosed the thing and was probably responsible for Tim's seizures. I watched through the observer's scope as he did a world-class job, then we booked it for the house. Everybody in the OR was giddy; Theresa turned on some terrible country and western music- I hate music in the OR- and we made record time closing. Gary woke Tim up as soon as we took him out of the pincers and he was stone cold normal, thank you Jesus.

Then I went out to talk to Momma. Not much mystery here, so I just told her like it happened. She was not pleased, even with a normal kid absent his cavernoma, and I could completely understand that. I understood it a little less well when two days later she signed Tim out AMA and the following Monday when she filed a malpractice suit claiming, "permanent disfigurement and possible irreversible brain damage."

I never saw Tim again- no clue who took out his stitches- and the University ultimately paid $35,000 to settle the suit, which if you know anything about medical malpractice litigation is a real bargain. I went home that night, hugged my two boys, kissed my wonderful wife and thought about how I had the best job in the entire world. Fuck a bunch of bikers.

My other regrettable personal experience with wrong side surgery involved a young partner of mine, a fantastic operative surgeon named Anthony, who was, and is, almost as pig-headed as he is smart. My dad, raised on a ranch in rural Canada, used to say about folks like Tony: "He's as independent as a hog on ice", a visual metaphor which captures Dr. Anthony's personality completely. At the time of this incident he was just out of training and had been with us for a couple of years; he was itching to show the world at large and me in particular he didn't need any help. That's a phase most surgeons pass through before coming to the realization we all need every bit of the help we can get and sometimes even that's not enough.

Anthony had a particular patient set up for surgery on a relatively routine, albeit quite large aneurysm located on the major branch of the right carotid artery at the brain's base, a case he could normally do skin-to-skin in about 2 1/2 hours. I had an early morning meeting that day but told him I'd come down to the OR around 1000, just to see how things were going. You would have thought I'd questioned his manhood.

"No way. I got this- I'll be done before you're out of that damn meeting, for sure."

Good enough. So, I spent most of the morning sitting on my ass listening to some administrative fool who hadn't seen a patient in 20 years tell us how we could make our practices more patient-friendly, the buzz word of that year. I'd heard the same bullshit in different words maybe 20 times before. Since I can't sleep sitting up, and my bad knee was bothering me, it was a semi-painful and very boring experience. Finally, I surreptitiously triggered my beeper, faked taking a call and then nodded apologetically, mouthing "it's the OR" and making my get-away. Just one of the many perks of being a surgeon- I mean, what are they going to say? "Don't go"?

I knew Tony would be long finished, with his patient back in the ICU, but since we ran three ORs that day, I figured I'd drop by to see what the other guys were doing, even though I had a TV monitor on my desk that would let me look at every room. The truth is, if you've spent your life as a surgeon, generally you love just being in the OR, any OR. You love the people, the camaraderie, the sense of purpose and mission, the whole damn thing. And if you're a part of a good team, it's even better.

So, I flash by Tony's OR on the way to see what my other partners are doing and much to my surprise I see that he's still operating. I wondered if for some reason, he'd gotten a late start. I knew for certain there wasn't a catastrophe underway, because I had an agreement with our long-serving neurosurgery nurses that if any of our surgeons got into serious trouble they were to page me immediately. I thought, "Well, what the hell?' and quietly walked through the scrub room to stand behind him and get myself oriented on the TV monitor.

Except it didn't happen. He had a large amount of the brain's blood vessels exposed, but I couldn't identify a single one. By this time in my career I'd done about 2500 aneurysm cases and there are only so many variations on the normal anatomy, but what I was seeing on the TV screen wasn't one I could recognize. I walked over to the view-box where the imaging studies were displayed; this was a routine vascular problem with no anatomical variants involved. I checked the patient ID. Well, at least we were operating on the correct human being.

My walking back to the microscope caused Anthony to turn around; he looked at me, shook his head and said "I can't find the damn thing. It's just not here. I've been looking for over an hour- the anatomy is completely fucked -up, but there's no goddamn aneurysm."

Long pause." Please wash your hands and have a look before I close her."

So, I'm at the scrub sink thinking we've got some kind of reportable case here, a woman with completely abnormal anatomy that looks normal on x-ray, when this quiet voice back in my parietal lobe says, "You are a total idiot – he's on the wrong side of the fucking head," to which I respond, "No way. The images show the aneurysm is on the right, the head is turned to the left, the incision is on the right, the bone flap is on the right, and the anatomy is all wrong. We're gonna take some pictures and write this sucker up."

"Wrong side."

"Screw you, smartass parietal lobe."

So, I sat down at the microscope, and rather than try to make sense out of the craziness down at the bottom of the wound, I decreased the scope's magnification, backed out the focus and started at the brain's surface to work my way through YSG's steps to ultimately expose the mis-named Circle of Willis. Actually a pentagon formed by the major arteries located at the junction of the brain stem and overlying cortex, its components supply essentially all of the brain with blood, and it's the location of 85% of all aneurysms.

In about thirty seconds it's obvious that Surgeon Anthony had skipped a couple of YSG's critical early steps, consequently bypassing the arteries on the patient's right side only to dissect out the blood vessels of the left hemisphere, none of which normally get exposed during an operation for this particular aneurysm. When he hadn't found the expected anatomy, Tony had continued to increase the magnification of the microscope which automatically and dramatically narrows the field of view.

As the crow flies, the difference between where he was and where he wanted to be was only 2 inches, but at the base of the brain, that's as good as a mile. Most importantly -since every surgeon gets lost at some time- he had no clue as to how to get found.

Getting up from the surgeon's chair, I broke it to him as gently as possible. His mistake had cost the patient a couple of extra hours of anesthetic time, but nothing else. It was a humbling experience, but young Dr. Anthony could use some humbling. It worked for about a week.

In light of this case I guess it's not surprising that wrong site-wrong side surgery hasn't been eliminated by institution of the Universal Protocol; the current best data suggest there are at least 4-5 surgical errors of this type on a daily basis in the US. If that's the case, just imagine what the numbers were previously. However, it's my belief that most surgical errors are neither so simple to classify nor so potentially easy to address, and as Dr Reason points out in his application of his theory of human error to medicine, often it's the most experienced, most skilled individuals who make them.

In 2012, I was called by a young neurosurgeon in San Antonio whom I knew to be well-trained and very conscientious. His patient was a young (mid-40s) local businessman who had developed the insidious onset of weakness in both lower extremities over a period of 18 months. The guy was active, a reasonable athlete who had found that he could no longer walk an entire 18 holes, had progressive difficulty controlling his snow skis, especially late in the day, and had switched his aerobic exercise of choice from jogging to walking, primarily because he "didn't feel stable."

A complete medical work-up had demonstrated a motor paraparesis of his lower extremities, a questionable sensory level at about T6 and pathological reflexes in both legs. A good quality CT of his spine hadn't shown much, but with contrast enhancement a vascular abnormality of the spinal cord above T6 was obvious. MR had confirmed the presence of an ovoid vascular mass with associated enlarged vessels; the mass was either in or on the dorsal aspect of the spinal cord.

This astute neurosurgeon, who had also done an endovascular fellowship, performed a spinal cord angiogram. On the phone he described an arterio-venous malformation of modest size in the cord with an associated venous varix, which accounted for the bulbous structure seen on MR. As a pre-op measure, the surgeon had attempted to embolize the feeding arteries to the AVM, but had been unable to introduce a catheter into either one. Consequently, he wanted to send the patient, whom I'll call Chris Cotton, to us for surgical removal of the malformation.

I met Chris and his wife in our out-patient clinic where I confirmed the findings on his neurologic exam and then sorted through the huge number of images they'd brought on a disc. I didn't think another shot at embolization was worth the risk, so I outlined a plan to open his spinal canal, find the abnormal vessels on the surface of the cord and then track them to the AVM and take it out. Once the AVM was gone the dilated vein should collapse and the mass distorting the spinal cord would be gone. I didn't think we'd need to open the cord and remove the mass, although it's possible to do that without producing permanent neurological injury if you're very careful and really lucky.

Well, it didn't happen that way. After exposing the entire surface of the cord, I couldn't find any abnormal vessels – none. The cord itself looked completely normal except being expanded in the classical snake-that-ate-the-rat fashion right at the level of the mass seen on imaging.

After a lot of dithering, I incised the exact center of the cord's surface and deepened the cut to about 2 mm., at which point I encountered the tense, pulsating vascular mass we'd seen on the angiogram. When I would attempt to gently work my way around the damn thing, the spinal cord evoked responses we were monitoring would taper off abruptly, meaning that routine electrical activity in the cord had ceased. When I'd stop dissecting, they would gradually return to almost but not quite normal. After several tries, the responses failed to come back at all. At least electrically, the spinal cord had stopped functioning.

So here I am; I've done a big, painful operation, failed to even see, much less treat, the pathology and according to our monitoring techniques, severely injured the already-wounded spinal cord. Like the song says, "you got to know when to fold them," so we closed up and went home.

Unfortunately, the only thing that worked that day was the monitoring; Chris awakened from anesthesia completely paralyzed from about the belly button on down. On his second post-operative day he showed us a twitch in one quadriceps, but it was really slow going there for a while. By the end of the first week he was almost back to the way he'd come to us, if you discounted the severe pain associated with having his back dissembled. Needless to say, he still had the problem he'd trusted us to fix.

What had gone wrong? We'd touched all the bases, followed all the rules and this wasn't even close to the first spinal cord AVM I'd operated, but it hadn't behaved like any of the 20 or so others. Maybe because it wasn't like the others; maybe... it wasn't even an AVM.

Every neuro-radiologist at our institution had reviewed the images and agreed with the diagnosis... except one. Dianne Mendel, a delightful lady trained in South Africa, had been away on vacation when Chris' images had been shown in conference. When I trudged over to her office with the discs she glanced at them, said she didn't have much to add but would look them over when she had time and call me back. About three hours later Dianne found me in the OR. Long story short, she thought Chris had a rare, very vascular tumor, not an AVM.

A week later, Howell Moran- my partner and the best cord tumor surgeon I've ever seen- took Chris back to the OR. Howell split his cord over a long length and gently shucked the tumor out completely. Chris again got worse post-operatively, but rapidly improved and was home within a week. One year later, he e-mailed me a video his wife had made on a ski run in Colorado; Chris looked better than most folks out there. It wasn't perfect, but pretty sweet.

This stuff is hard, even when you're trying, and there aren't enough people like Chris... or Dianne.

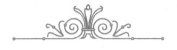

CHAPTER FIFTEEN

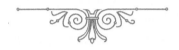

Mass Casuality

A mass casualty incident is simply defined as an event where the number and severity of casualties overwhelms the capability of emergency responders to manage them appropriately. By varying the number and severity of casualties and the capabilities of the initial responders, it's easy to see this definition can cover a broad spectrum of situations, making the application of the term to a specific event of questionable value. However, almost everybody in the lay or medical public would agree that the crash of a commercial airliner qualifies without question. During my practice, we dealt with two such crashes at Dallas-Fort Worth International airport within a period of three years. Let me tell you about one of them.

On 2 August 1985, Delta Flight 1109, a Lockheed 1011 Tristar airliner inbound to DFW from Ft. Lauderdale with 135 passengers and 11 crew members was caught during its final approach by a powerful wind shear more than a mile north of Runway 11-L. The big aircraft was first slammed to the ground and then into two huge water tanks. At the second collision the fuselage of the aircraft erupted in flame, breaking into two sections before coming to rest. One hundred twelve passengers and eight crewmembers would die either immediately or over the next twenty-four hours; essentially all of the victims, both dead and alive, were transported to Metropolitan Memorial Hospital where two more would die within the next six weeks.

Our neurosurgery team was finishing a routine workday at about 4 PM when the hospital was notified of the crash and the impending arrival of an unknown number of survivors. It's uncommon for a hospital to have the advantage of advance notice of a disaster of this magnitude, a forewarning that allows for the mobilization of both material and personnel. All available nursing and medical staff were requested to report to their normal duty stations, security resources were increased and control of all beds was centralized in the administrative core. Staffing in the Emergency Room was doubled and all non- emergency diagnostic procedures in the Radiology department were cancelled.

On a more granular level, the neurosurgery service assembled its resources in the eight-bed NICU and began to marshal forces. On deck were five fully-trained neurosurgeons, ten residents at various levels of training, two surgery interns fresh from medical school and a couple of visiting medical students. By the time we got around to counting heads in the ICU there were ten critical care nurses onsite with a couple of more on their way in, five LVNs and two ward clerks (secretaries). The ICU at that moment was caring for six patients, four of whom we could and did quickly transfer to our open floor, where they joined 18 other post-operative patients in good condition. We thought we were pretty fat, but actually had no clue what was coming.

Brain and spine trauma is, as a rule, not as labor-intensive, at least on the physician level, as major abdominal, chest or orthopedic trauma, for the simple reason that there's not that much tissue to injure and, once injured, there's less manpower needed to manage each injury. On the other hand, brain trauma especially is a time-critical phenomena; you better fix it quick if you plan to fix it at all. So, we reserved one empty OR with two designated surgeons on strip alert (meaning in the Surgeons' Lounge) and two circulating nurses primed and ready to go; our scrub nurse was scrubbed, gowned and gloved with a craniotomy instrument set open and a spine set on the back table. Because of the late hour, a second empty OR was available to be designated for neurosurgical use if and when the need arose.

Tim Lord, our chief resident about whom you'll hear more, was stationed down in the PIT with one of his junior colleagues to manage acute care and triage (a word derived from the French verb meaning to sort); these two were backed up by two surgery teams (each composed of a faculty surgeon plus a resident). Because almost all modern neurosurgery is based on imaging findings, both teams were stationed immediately adjacent to the Emergency Room in the Radiology department; they would accompany any critically injured patients directly to the operating suite or to the ICU if necessary. It's difficult to overestimate the risks involved with transferring brain or spine -injured patients from stretchers to OR or Radiology tables and we didn't plan on hurting anybody in transit. Our remaining troops were divided between our routine ward and the NICU. Another significant risk in mass casualty management is the tendency to overlook patients already under one's care in all the excitement of the new arrivals. My role was just to be where ever we needed another opinion or a second set of hands.

The first ambulances began to arrive at the ER's loading dock around 6 PM; we caught our initial admission from the second group of patients. This young woman, on her way from Florida to L.A., was incoherent on examination and had to be restrained to keep her on the examination table. About the sole piece of information that could be initially ascertained was that her neck hurt. The Trauma surgeons (lords of the ER) swarmed around her for about fifteen minutes, at the end of which we were assured that systemically she had no obvious injuries and that she was sufficiently stable as to undergo imaging. She remained uncooperative and confused, so using the ample IV access Trauma had provided, we cautiously gave her a small dose of diazepam. She quieted down almost immediately to the extent that Tim could perform a detailed neurological exam; he found she was exquisitely tender in the mid-portion of her neck, as well as being slightly weak in both arms. To a neurosurgeon, this is a spinal cord injury until proven otherwise, so, within about 20 minutes of her arrival, she was in hard cervical collar in the CT scanner under the surveillance of the first neurosurgery back-up team.

Because of her confusion, we coupled the obligatory cervical spine study with a quick brain scan. The studies identified a very small cortical contusion which would bear watching and a much more important fracture -dislocation between the fifth and sixth cervical vertebrae. This would account for her bilateral arm weakness and would require surgical stabilization; however because of her young age and slender body habitus, Tim felt the dislocation could possibly be reduced with gentle distraction. He handed her off to the back-up team and went back into the PIT just as two more ambulances arrived. The patient was placed in our first set of cervical tongs; with a little more diazepam she relaxed enough that her fracture reduced itself. Within five minutes her arm strength began to return and her neck pain to subside. Not knowing what more compelling misery was in the pipeline, her two neurosurgeons escorted her up to the NICU to await a delayed operation, and the second back-up team stepped up.

The ambulances just kept coming. There were a smattering of other injuries- chest, belly, arm and leg- but the majority of patients were badly burned. Metropolitan Memorial has a world-famous burn unit, and those guys and girls were all over the ER that night and into the following morning. The care of burn victims is perhaps the most "hands-on" of anything in medicine including the management of complete spinal cord injury patients. These injured folks were literally covered up with physicians and nurses struggling to deal with their pain, shock, compromised airways, burned and blistered extremities, seared faces and singed hair. The smell of burned flesh flooded the big ER and spilled out into the hallways.

By this time we caught our second patient, again with neck pain but this time with numbness and tingling in both hands, a bright warning light came on. Immediately, our so-called "index of suspicion" went through the roof, and we started to look at everyone in the ER as a probable cervical spine injury. Now, we obnoxiously insisted that even the badly-burned patients undergo a neck x-ray before being transferred to the Burn ICU; sure enough, one was found to have an unstable spine fracture and a second had a stable "chip" fracture, probably of no clinical significance. That young man was also placed in tongs -which would not interfere with the treatment of his burns- and his name entered on our "To Do" list. Of the twenty-two survivors, ultimately eight were proven to have suffered neck fractures that night and a final patient was identified the following day, a bad oversight on admission that could, but did not have, serious consequences.

The initial management of cervical spinal column injuries involves stabilizing the spine with the use of a traction device known as Gardner-Wells tongs. This little life-saver consists of a thin semi-circular metal frame threaded at each end by a spring-loaded, calibrated screw which itself is tipped by an extremely sharp pin. When the frame, which looks like a skinny horseshoe with spikes on each end, is placed correctly on a patient's head so that it encircles the skull, the pins encounter the scalp just above the tip of the external ear on both sides. This location marks the central axis of rotation of the neck and is generally the correct direction of distraction to eliminate or reduce dislocation of the vertebrae. Once the sites of insertion are identified, the skin there is anesthetized with an injectable local anesthetic and then the pins are literally screwed into the underlying skull. Sounds gruesome, but it's almost painless and incredibly effective.

Within the first hour, we'd exhausted the hospital's inventory of cervical spine tongs, and facing an unknown but potentially large number of additional spine-injured patients we needed at least ten more sets, right now. Fortunately, the entire population of North Texas was glued to television broadcasts of the disaster, so communication with the other major hospitals wasn't a big problem, and almost immediately we had seven dispatch riders, with police escorts, on the road.

An hour after recognizing our potential shortage, we were sterilizing 12 borrowed sets of GW tongs. It's a given that when dealing with borrowed medical equipment, at least 10% won't work, but with a little fiddling we had ten functional sets, all of which we ended up using. To my knowledge, this was the only shortage the hospital encountered throughout the next week; in part that's grim testimony to the unfortunately small number of individuals who survived the initial crash.

Of twenty-two people that made it to the hospital alive, nine had broken necks, an unexpected testimony to the violent and sudden deceleration forces brought to bear on the neck when the head is unsupported. Fortunately, only two of our patients with broken necks-the initial two- had spinal cord injuries; these were mild and reversible once their spinal columns were placed back in alignment, even prior to being fused surgically.

A second unexpected consequence of that extreme flexion-extension is the internal disruption of one or both carotid arteries ("carotid dissection") in the neck, a process that shears off the internal lining of the artery and can produce either immediate or delayed strokes. Seven patients were found to have this complication, and unfortunately, two of these suffered stroke-like symptoms before we recognized the source of the problem. All seven patients underwent emergent repair or replacement of the damaged arteries either on the evening of admission or early the following morning. Ironically none of these patients had injuries to the vertebral arteries which actually traverse the bony wings of the vertebra in their route to the brain.

Surgical repairs of carotid dissections are really sweet operative procedures that have almost completely been replaced in the last ten years by the development of techniques to repair the ruptured interior of the artery using catheter-deployed stents. Back in the day, an extensive length of the carotid system was exposed via a longitudinal neck incision, following which the dissected portion of the artery was identified, clamped off and removed. Meanwhile a second surgical team exposed the saphenous venous system in the patient's leg and removed an appropriate length of the vein, resecting its valves so as not to impede blood flow or to promote clot formation. Then, using intravenous heparin the patient was anti-coagulated and the venous graft sutured in place to replace the injured artery. The heparin was then "reversed"- meaning its anti-coagulant effects nullified by a second medication – the graft checked for flow and any leaks promptly repaired before the wound was closed.

Seven of these operations going on in two adjacent ORs, coupled with several orthopedic cases and two neurosurgery spine procedures kept things hopping; none of the several burn patients would undergo surgery until they were stabilized, which required at least 48 hours.

So, it was a long night. The most surprising news was that we treated only one significant head injury that required surgery; this was a young man with a depressed fracture of his skull which must have occurred either at the time of impact or perhaps as he tried to exit the aircraft. He'd suffered a brief loss of consciousness and was amnestic for the time period around the crash, but aside from a bloody laceration, he was neurologically intact in the PIT. He subsequently got a quick, clean surgical procedure early that following morning, and was ready for discharge to his home in California two days later.

By 5:00 AM -11 hours after the first patient's arrival-the furor was pretty much over, at least for those of us in neurosurgery. We had four new admissions in our ICU plus one in the Burn ICU, had done three operations (two spine, one head) with two more on hold, and I'd scrubbed on two of the Vascular Surgery operations for people with dissected carotids. We'd started releasing our nursing staff a couple of hours earlier but wouldn't go to the regular physician on-call schedule until about 7 AM.

I swung through the PIT and radiology just to be sure there was no hanging chad, then peeked into the NICU, where everything was calm. That was in contrast to the controlled chaos of the Burn Unit, where I gowned and gloved before being allowed to check the tongs on our cervical spine injuries. The attending surgeon told me he had "no idea" when either patient would be cleared for a spine operation, and I nodded in reply.

"As long as your nurses kept the pin sites clean, those tongs can stay in place forever. We'll just keep checking on them but let us be the ones to tighten the screws if they need it. I don't want to have to take one of those pins out of either one's temporal lobe."

One of the patients was a young man in previously good health; I thought there was an excellent chance his fracture would heal without surgery long before the Burn docs would clear him for operation, but we could sort that out down the road. The other, suffering from an extensive burn injury, was in critical condition and at best weeks away from an elective spine procedure.

The big trauma hospital is joined to the medical school's office building by a multi-floored, glass – enclosed walkway, which opens out in front with a view over the main entrance. In the back, the more modest glass windows look down on a confluence of parking lots and a small two-story brick laboratory that houses the County Medical Examiner's Office. As I walked across the passageway on the way to my office, my eyes were drawn to activity in the parking area where there were multiple large tractor-trailer units being pulled into a ordered formation centered on the ME's building. Stopping, I counted 10 long trailers, with an additional two idling on the adjacent street . All of the trucks seemed to have their motors running. Because of the angle of my view, it was impossible to make out the identity of any of the parked units, but the two refrigerated vans on the street were easy to recognize, as was the County logo stenciled on their sides. One hundred and twenty dead people need a lot of storage space. That sobering realization made for a long ride home.

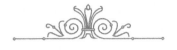

CHAPTER SIXTEEN

Road Games

Neurosurgery as practiced in the so-called Second and Third Worlds is not a mystery to American neurosurgeons, as many of us from both academic and private communities travel abroad to teach, evaluate patients, and often to perform surgical procedures. Regardless of the sponsoring agencies, which range from university exchanges, medical missions, and professional conferences to 'special" private arrangements, these working trips are almost always win-win propositions. The host country benefits by the importation and dissemination of medical talent and expertise, while the American visitors relish the opportunity to reach out to new patient populations, to teach new 'tricks' to appreciative audiences and to learn about the practice of their chosen specialty in a new and often distinctly difference environment.

Being an invited "visitor" involves fulfilling a different role from that of a contract employee of the local government or an NGO like Médecins Sans Frontiers. Exactly what a visiting surgeon is permitted to do on these expeditions is variable; in most situations, a visitor's professional activity is dependent on two factors: the first being the visitor's professional reputation and the second, the degree of sophistication of the host medical system. If the traveling neurosurgeon is a world renown expert with special skills, even the US may let him do his thing after jumping through a gauntlet of hoops, whereas in the most primitive medical societies, all a visitor may need to obtain unlimited operative privileges is a printed copy of his invitation and his business card.

Although a significant portion of my surgical training took place in France and Switzerland, most of my foreign operating experience was obtained in South America, where our department conducted a periodic series of educational trips and where I subsequently made several solo visits, usually to operate on specific patients with cerebro-vascular diagnoses. As a group, we got started on these 'medical missions" through the efforts of a retired Colombian-American neurosurgeon named Listo Puerto, who was the first neurosurgery resident to be trained in our own program.

Listo came to our Medical Center in 1962 after completing four years of surgical training in Colombia; he spent three years with us, satisfying the requirements of the American Board of Neurological Surgery in 1965. After passing his Board Examinations, rather than return to Colombia, Listo set up practice in Bedford Texas, almost equidistant between Dallas and Ft. Worth. He recruited a series of several partners, had a successful practice for over 15 years and then retired to spend half his time in Texas and the remaining six months of each year in Barranquilla, Colombia where he and his wife Lora bought a beautiful home. Listo, a Barranquilla homeboy, remained involved with the neurosurgery community there after his retirement, teaching at the local medical school and ultimately sponsoring several young surgeons to come to Dallas for brief periods as observers.

In the early 1990s, Listo began to pester me about creating a jointly-sponsored educational mission that would take several of our surgeons to Columbia to lecture and to provide some "operative demonstrations.' He independently obtained over 50% of the necessary funding from the Colombian Society of Neurosurgeons; with that money in hand and a detailed plan, the two of us were able to convince our own university to sanction the trip and to tote the rest of the note.

Listo's idea was to have a group of 4-6 surgeons travelling to selected medical schools, seeing patients, giving talks and operating on specific cases in different venues around Colombia. The basic plan was to spend two days in each facility, the first for lecturing and the second day for surgery. Our initial trip was planned for four days on the ground plus a travel day on each end; our first hosts were to be the medical school faculties in Cartagena and Listo's home town of Barranquilla, both located on the Caribbean coast in the far Northwest of Colombia.

Listo was responsible for all the Colombian ground work, while the approval process on our end was limited to obtaining legal disclaimers insuring that the great State of Texas, the Medical Center and its employees were indemnified against charges of death, disability, malfeasance and other damages we might inflict while on the road. Our end of things took over 15 months to straighten out; meanwhile Dr. Puerto was hustling from city to city, medical school to medical school, establishing dates, securing lecture venues, making inter-city travel arrangements, reserving lodging and, not least of all, finding us some patients to fix.

When I went over all these steps with Listo on multiple occasions he repeatedly assured me the last item was the least problematic. "Duke, my boy- patients is what we got lots of. We got more patients every day than your whole department could operate in a whole damn year. Sicker patients in our parking lots than you got in the ICU."

Listo was easy to believe; he had an iron-clad reputation for living up to what he said. Just one example will make the point. As a resident, the Neurosurgery Residents' call room, where he actually lived full-time, was on the ward at Metro Memorial shared by Neurosurgery and Thoracic Surgery. One particular evening, the patient care room across the hall was occupied by a completely inebriated trauma patient with multiple rib fractures who screamed at full volume with every breath. Listo complained to the thoracic surgery resident, but all the chest cutter would promise was that his service planned on doing a tracheostomy on the screamer after he had sobered up the following day. Listo shook his head:" If you boys don't do something about this, I will."

The screaming stopped abruptly about 1 AM, and when the thoracic surgeons made rounds six hours later, they realized the scheduled procedure had already been accomplished. By then Listo was down in the operating suite, ready for the first neurosurgery case.

Our visit as initially scheduled entailed lectures at the local medical schools, operations at various University Hospitals and social events at a variety of faculty and private clubs. At that time in Colombia, in-patient health care was divided between not-for-profit hospitals, such as those sponsored primarily by religious organizations, smaller "private "clinics exclusively for paying clientele and large" University Hospitals", government -funded institutions for the large medically indigent population.

The medical staffs at the University Hospitals were physicians in training. Their supervision was variable, ranging from slight to invisible, but these large "charity" facilities were teeming with what physicians refer to as "great pathology", meaning a vast array of disease conditions thus far untouched by modern medicine. As such, they were potentially fertile training grounds for hungry young surgeons… and ideal venues places for visiting firemen to strut their stuff.

Listo's initial plan was to divide our visiting surgical team in half, with one group lecturing all day and the other working in various operating rooms, then to switch the order the following day. Like all good plans, this one fell apart at first sight of the enemy, but actually each of our five surgeons ultimately did spend at least three days doing procedures, and Dr. Rafe Green, the sole neurologist on the trip, stayed busy between hospitals, looking in on our pre- and post-op patients, showing the Colombians the ropes with some new anti-convulsant medications, and serving as an on-the-spot translator. Rafe and Listo were old buddies whose training in Dallas had over-lapped by a year; they shared a weird version of Spanglish that a surprising number of both Americans and Colombians understood. Organizationally, the two of them were priceless is dealing with the quasi-diplomatic bureaucracy that encased our visit.

Our other surgical pilgrims were Dale Smith, a crackerjack pediatric surgeon, Howell Moran -our spine surgery guru- Bryce Michaels who specialized in tumor and seizure surgery, and Henry Baylor, who like me was a vascular neurosurgeon. In Colombia, our routine day started about 8, with breakfast in the hotel, after which we'd scatter out across the landscape to our appointed hospitals or lecture venues. Generally, we'd get back to the hotel in the neighborhood of 7 PM for a shower, cocktails and a late dinner and /or social event every night. For me at least, the real highlight of our trip was the late night bull sessions, generally in my room, where, lubricated with good Colombian beer, we'd hot-wash that day and plan for the next.

In the two weeks prior to our arrival in Colombia, the US government had unexpectedly tossed a monkey wrench into our travel schedule by announcing a unilateral intensification of "the war on drugs" with a special focus on Colombia, where the US claimed the local government wasn't pulling its share of the enforcement load. The official rhetoric went something like "unless Colombia gets with the program, foreign aid would be drastically reduced and Colombian travel to the States would be severely restricted". This rude shock produced some real problems for our modest plans to travel merrily around the country.

After our arrival, road blocks -complete with body searches -suddenly were everywhere; coming in on a later flight than the other team members, I was stopped twice between the airport and the city. There was an understandable Colombian reflex to make Americans caught in the clamp-down uncomfortable, so, every time we went outside our hotel, our medical convoy was stopped at least once. During these stops random members of the group would be thoroughly frisked, usually by a teenaged National Guardsman overseen by a second teenager, distractedly waving a loaded M16. Our hosts grew sufficiently concerned with safety that ultimately, they deleted potential visits to Bogota and Medellin from our schedule.

During the week, our five surgeons did a reasonable number of serious procedures. Dale operated some kids with congenital deformities and did a nasty brain tumor, Bryce took out a couple of complex tumors of the posterior fossa plus a brain abscess and Howell did some simple spine reconstructions and a cord tumor. None of these cases, in and of themselves, were extraordinarily difficult; consequently our multiple Colombian observers were politely appreciative, but not overwhelmed by the chops of the boys from Dallas. That said, these were all "away" games, in strange environments with unfamiliar assistants who knew nothing of our routines, etc. We were regularly introduced to a startling assortment of neurosurgical instruments (some of which I'd only seen in medical history books) and much of the instrumentation on the nurses' back tables I didn't recognize at all. Of course, each of us had brought our own "go-to" stuff", the five or six tools we just couldn't do without, but for everything else we were at the mercy of the local customs. To complicate matters further, almost none of the scrub nurses spoke any English, so the going was a little rocky at the start.

As Henry and I were doing our first case, I turned to the observers (all full-fledged neurosurgeons from the local community) and suggested that one of the local neurosurgeons might want to help by scrubbing and translating for the scrub tech. You would have thought I'd insulted the manhood of the entire guild of Colombian neurosurgery; a surgeon working as a nurse? After an embarrassing silence- and no volunteers- we compromised by the Americans initially scrubbing in pairs, one doing the cutting and the other helping the scrub look for instruments. Thankfully the nurses caught on to our routines quickly and we each picked up some Spanish nomenclature as well, so by Day Three we were rocking and rolling.

Day Three, our first in Cartagena, was the day Henry and I headed out to the local University Hospital to fix a ruptured aneurysm. We'd looked at the angiograms the previous evening (pretty routine large anterior communicating aneurysm) and learned a little about the patient (early 40s, good health, 1st hemorrhage, in good neurological condition, now about 10 days post-bleed). So we loaded up our special stuff, to include a selection of aneurysm clips from home, and joined a mini-caravan of five cars (one Mercedes, two Land Cruisers and a couple of new Tahoes) filled with local neurosurgeons for the trip through the old city to the hospital campus. We were only stopped once. The Guardsmen opened all our instrument packs and threatened to confiscate our aneurysm clips (no, gentlemen- not silver, just titanium) which would have really been a bummer, but Listo finally talked them into taking the hotel's picnic lunch instead, and we made it to the University Hospital about an hour late.

The hospital itself most resembled a medium-security prison built about 1880 using cinder blocks and concrete, but it sat in a pleasant park-like setting just off the city's main drag. Perhaps I thought "park-like" because there were tents pitched everywhere with people out on the grass doing everything from taking a leak to washing their laundry. I looked over at Listo, who muttered, "Families of the patients." No shit.

Inside, the hospital lived up to its exterior promise. Colombia is a warm country, but interior climate control was limited to a scattering of window units and a vast array of ceiling fans. The "patient-care spaces", meaning the wards, were huge, open, and sweltering (much like our own city-county hospitals in 1967); on the elevator ride up to the OR Suite, Listo assured me the individual ORs were air- conditioned. That's important for reasons a lot more critical than the surgeons' comfort: it's often very difficult to maintain a patient's normal body temperature during prolonged general anesthesia, a problem which can have a profound effect on issues like cardiac and kidney function, clotting mechanisms and respiration, just to mention a few.

Once through the main OR doors we were shown to a dressing room with open lockers complete with scrubs, caps, masks and booties. When we were suited up and had given our valuables to one of the local neurosurgeons (who carried them around in a bag), the OR director herded all fourteen of us down the hall to the NS operating room. Parked just outside the door was a gurney- a hospital stretcher on wheels- and parked on the gurney were two dudes, both dressed in scrubs, sharing a smoke. One of them was introduced as our anesthetist for the morning; the other was our patient. Because of the small butterfly needle in the back of his right hand, he couldn't shake hands, but we got a grin.

With Listo's help and a lot of hand motions, we tried to explain to our prospective victim just exactly what we'd planned for him. His face reflected exactly zero interest as he watched Henry pantomime sawing his head open, moving his brain around and clipping this bad blood vessel that had made him sick. When we both ran out of gas, the guy looked over at Listo and said, "Bueno." So much for informed consent.

The operation was sort of anti-climactic, but the OR itself was not. About 20' x 30', it featured a ragged hole that had been pounded in one concrete wall to fit a small window air conditioner. The unit sounded like a 100cc two stroke dirt bike permanently stuck in second gear, but it produced a focal wave of cooler air which was channeled in the general direction of the patient's body through a tunnel formed by sheets draped on IV poles. Nonetheless, with the patient, the gas passer, the scrub and circulating nurses, Listo and his 11 local friends, the two of us surgeons and one guy (Roberto) who had just showed up to do the hard work of getting us in the head, all packed in this closed space, it was hotter than hell. No time to fool around.

After Henry and I turned the skin flap and sketched out the desired bony opening on the bare skull, our buddy Roberto brought out his magical drill. This thing was about the size of a small jack hammer and looked like it had been put together in high school auto shop class, but it damn sure could make holes; when Roberto changed out the drill bit for the saw blade (which had no guard) you could see the guy was a master. He cut the sweetest bone flap exactly where Henry had traced the incision in 15 seconds flat. Then, as icing on the cake, he popped up the flap with the saw blade, catching it in the air with his off hand.

I said, "Que bueno!" He bowed slightly at the waist, dropped the drill on a side table, gave the bone flap to the scrub and left the room. He'd be back for the closure.

Henry, who'd played some serious baseball, said," That guy's got one hell of a heater."

Once the dura was open, we were ready to pull the microscope in and get down to business. The scope itself was an older, basic model without bells or whistles, but the optics were fine. What wasn't fine was the sterilization procedure for the body, frame and associated electrical cords: as in, there wasn't any. In the US, Asia and Europe, microscopes are carefully draped in sterile plastic sheaths that prevent the surgeon's gloved hands from touching the non-sterile surfaces of the scope, stand and cords, then inadvertently contaminating the open wound or the surgical instruments. Here in the University Hospital, the scrub nurse just took a small alcohol sponge and casually went over the microscope before pushing it into place, then looking up as if to say, "It's all yours, bigshot."

Henry, the perpetual smartass, muttered in my ear, "In the States this is what we call "bareback."

During a brain surgery procedure being done with a basic microscope, the spectators can't see a damned thing. A monocular assistant's eyepiece which can be adjusted to coincide with the surgeon's view is loosely attached to the main body, but in the oldest models- which this definitely was- the viewing tube must have its focus continually adjusted manually to match the surgeon's focus and at best the tube shows only a portion of the surgeon's field of view. Modern OR set-ups compensate by substituting a beam splitter attachment feeding into a small TV camera whose output is projected on one or multiple screens around the OR or even to remote locations. Needless to say, here we had just the monocular tube, which the eleven visitors queued up to use, each with no qualms about vigorously adjusting the focus.

Repetitive movement of the monocular tube jostles the surgeon's eyepieces so as to make their use impossible and since every time one of these bozos took a peek, he had to communicate his impressions to the rest of the room, what we had there at the head of the OR table could best be described as a "chaotic situation totally inimical to safe, effective brain surgery" otherwise known as a complete cluster-fuck. After about three minutes- a full rotation of the 11 observers- I grew to appreciate the hopelessness of the situation, and in about twenty more seconds I'd secured everyone's undivided attention. Every Colombian I could see looked terribly embarrassed, so I took a deep breath, apologized, and we started again with a little better mutual understanding of the ground rules.

Fortunately, this was a straight-forward anterior communicating artery aneurysm that almost completely exposed itself with very minimal sharp dissection. Once it was hanging out in the breeze, I climbed out of the surgeon's chair and invited every mother's son to have a long look through the surgeon's eyepieces. Then, still playing cultural catch-up after my outburst, I asked each man to offer his educated input as to how best to clip the damn thing. An impromptu conference produced consensus that a left-handed clip placement would be optimal, so I asked Henry- a native southpaw- if he'd do the honors while I switched to play-by-play.

My partner sat down, hammed it up pretty good, changed his clip selection twice and then nailed it.

Everybody relaxed, but when he asked the scrub nurse for a long spinal needle, the crowd got nervous and held its breath. There was a little gasp as he perforated the aneurysm sac, but being safely and completely sealed off from the artery by the clip, the bulging blister just shriveled up. I could hear the crowd's sigh of relief. Having proven the thing was defused, Henry turned around for our ritual high five and we started to close.

The crowd began to move sort of rhythmically: over my left shoulder I could see our hosts (all 11) high- fiving one another. I winked at Henry who just shook his head, and fortunately, about then our old friend Roberto and some other dude showed up for the closure. So, soaked with sweat, we bowed out and retired to the dressing room for some ice water with sliced lemons.

Neither Henry nor I ever saw our patient again, but Listo assured us "the poor guy did just fine."

Unfortunately, road games sometimes don't end with high fives all around and we-beat-the-devil-stories over drinks back at the hotel. If you're playing a high stakes contest in unfamiliar territory and things go to hell in a handbasket, it's just the naked 'expert'- no supportive team, no familiar instruments, no faithful anesthetist- against the badness, and the badness always gets a vote.

About a year after our first Colombian trip we went back for an encore; more stops, more lectures, more surgeries. Our team had changed a little but was still anchored on our two heavy hitters, Bryce and Howell, and we still had Listo running interference, so at the end of a busy week we flew out of Cartagena without any patient or doctor casualties, except for some GI distress that kept me running up and down the aisle most of the flight from Colombia to Miami.

On our next-to-last day, I'd operated a young woman with a small AVM located on the surface of a "non- eloquent" part of the brain called the cerebellum. She'd had a single hemorrhage, was in great condition and the bleed had made a little cavity just deep to the malformation, so the AVM was almost dangling out in the breeze. We operated the patient in one of the larger private hospitals which had a nice scope set-up with good TV projection; all in all, it was a good teaching case. Joaquin Rodriquez, the young Colombian neurosurgeon who was assisting me, was obviously good enough to be one of our own, so I mostly provided suggestions and narration to the crowd while he took the thing out in fine style. The proverbial piece of cake.

That evening at the dinner to mark the end of our visit, I was introduced to a senior neurosurgeon -cum- politician, el Doctor Segovia, who later invited me out on the patio for cigars. This was prior to my femur fracture and I was a real aficionado, so I readily accepted his invitation to enjoy what turned out to be a couple of sweet Cuban Macanudos. Cigars are definitely an acquired and sinful taste; I haven't had one now in 15 years, but they're a well-remembered pleasure and sometimes can form a nice bridge from social chit-chat to more serious professional conversation.

It turned out Dr. Segovia had a patient, a young woman with a "worrisome AVM, almost a mirror image of today's case", although she had not suffered a hemorrhage but rather had increasingly severe headaches. He thought that her future was "perilous" but had up to this point been reluctant to recommend surgical treatment. Today's case had given him second thoughts. What, might he ask, was my opinion?

So, I'm a brain surgeon that specializes in vascular diseases. At this point in my career I'd operated on a little over 400 AVM patients and managed to maintain my optimism despite having had "poor results" (defined as dead or disabled) in 11% of my cases. What did the guy expect? I said I'd be interested in looking at the patient and her images, but if the situation was actually similar to today's patient, all other things being equal, surgery would probably beat the lady's chances of living with the malformation for the next 50 years.

The caveat obviously was two-fold; in the realm of human diseases all things are rarely equal, and surgical results, especially in complex problems like arterio-venous malformations, depend on one hell of a lot more than the casual impressions of a tired surgeon with two drinks in him who has never laid eyes on either the patient or her x-rays.

El Doctor gave me a grin, another Macanudo and a big abrazo. He said he'd be in touch.

Back in Dallas, things were really busy. Henry had moved to the upper Midwest to become the chief of neurosurgery at a famous medical center, and we'd brought on a tremendously talented young surgeon named Thomas to share the growing volume of cerebrovascular diseases. I didn't think much about Colombia again until some six months later when I received a long letter from el Doctor Segovia formally inviting me to return to operate on the young patient he'd described to me previously. He suggested a series of potential dates for my visit, outlined a plan of reimbursement for my travel expenses and detailed a compensation proposal he requested I submit to our business office. Dr. Segovia also sent some additional medical records, including a radiologist's report of the patient's diagnostic angiogram, which made this AVM sound like more of a surgical challenge that the previous case, but it also sounded like the radiologist didn't have a real clue about his business. The angiogram itself was not included.

One of the many nice things about being employed by a University-based health system was the lack of hassle about patient billing. The actual prices for surgical procedures were established by the system itself with reference to the Medicare standards, while the billing and collecting was done by the University's financial office. I worked for a generous salary that was related in part to my surgical receipts, in part to my academic jobs of clinical research and teaching and in part to my administrative duties as the chairman of a busy surgical department. I never, in almost forty years of practice, discussed financial charges with a patient, and generally didn't know what the bill for my services would be. So, I was a little taken back by Segovia's offer to collect for my surgery. After talking with the financial troops, we decided the best thing would be to treat this just like one of the cases I'd done on our official Colombian visits; there wouldn't be a surgical bill, at least not from me. The only thing the medical school insisted on was the legal disclaimer.

The administrative to-and- fro took a couple of months this time; finding a four-day soft spot in my schedule took another three. All in all, about six months after Segovia had invited me, I was preparing to go to the airport for the trip when my new partner Tony wandered into my office, sprawled out on my couch and said he'd like to see the angiogram of this AVM I was flying down to Central America to fix. I was mildly embarrassed to admit that I'd only just received an abbreviated version of what was a very substandard arteriogram, which nevertheless suggested that this was anything but a mirror image of the "piece of cake" case. I put the few films I did have up on my view box, and he leaned over for a quick peek. Since I'd spent the last couple of years drumming the need for proper preparation into his former Marine skull, I wasn't surprised when he looked back at me as if my fly was open. Getting up, Dr. Anthony wandered back out the door, saying over his shoulder, "I hope you know something about this case that I don't."

It was a wake-up call. Now, I had two choices: #1- trust what I'd been told and get on the plane: #2-be a hard ass and cancel the trip until somebody in Colombia got their shit together and either sent me all the images, or did a new, complete angiogram and sent that. A third choice- make the trip but don't commit to the operation – didn't seem fair to anyone involved. Looked at objectively, what was at stake here wasn't money, reputation or inconvenience; it was this young lady's life. That's always the bottom line, but that day I failed to frame the question in that stark fashion. I went.

By the time I got off the airplane the wheels were in motion. I would go directly from the airport to meet the patient and her family in Dr. Segovia's office; the following morning I'd review all the images (finally), visit the OR to go over my operative plan with the anesthetist and nursing staff, then talk a final time with the patient after her admission to hospital that evening. Then would come the operative day, followed by one post-op day on the ground; my return to Texas was scheduled on the fourth morning. A pretty tight schedule with very little room for complications; tough AVMs are notorious for complications. And as it turned out, this was a tough AVM; when I looked at the actual angiogram films, its resemblance to the previous case ended with them both being in roughly the same part of the brain. In fact, the angiogram showed this AVM was three times the size of the "piece of cake" case, had feeding from four of the six major arteries of the cerebellum and had one extension that went right down to, but didn't enter, the brain stem. It would be a tough case back home, and that's where I should have gone the following day. When push comes to shove, regardless of every other consideration, the only thing that counts is what's best for the patient.

The next afternoon, after seven hours of operation and six units of blood my patient was still stable; the nurses had done yeomen's work and the funky-looking anesthetist had played his role like a pro, but I could see there way no way I was going to untangle what was left of this AVM from this young girl's brain stem. Thus far, I didn't think I'd hurt her, but if I pushed it any farther I would run the dual risks of injuring her brain stem and loosing control of the arterial input, meaning possible bleeding that I wouldn't be able to control. So, I took a five-minute break, spent most of it cursing myself for ever even thinking about putting her in this position, then told everyone the party was over- I was baling out.

We closed slowly and very carefully, watching her blood pressure like hawks. When by accident or intent you fail to remove the entire AVM, the remainder is "unstable", meaning very prone to hemorrhage, especially in the early hours after operation. And, as far as we understand, that elevated risk persists for the remainder of the patient's life.

After we had the girl safely bedded down in the Recovery Ward I talked to her family at length. Instead of being outraged that I hadn't done what I'd been brought three thousand miles to do, they were elated that she'd lived through the operation and that I'd "removed most of the AVM," which I honestly told them did nothing to reduce her chance of hemorrhage in the future. In fact, it may well have made a bleed more likely. I couldn't even convince Dr. Segovia, who just patted me on the back, said I'd done a "fine job" and gave me a couple of his Macanudos. I felt like shit, went back to the hotel and called my wife to tell her she was married to a gutless idiot. She remined me she'd known about the "idiot" part for a while, but thought I was still a keeper and should get some sleep. There're really no surprises for trauma surgeons; they know all about having your ass handed to you by a bad case.

The kid still looked good the following morning and her arteriogram done early that afternoon showed about a tenth of the original malformation was still filling with blood, but even that flow was very slow. Segovia told the family he thought the thing might "clot off" by itself; complete bullshit which never happens. I told the family that either we needed to bring the girl to the US for a second operation or have the remnant irradiated by a special technique I knew could be done in Buenos Aires. They were so happy I hadn't maimed their daughter that they "wanted to think about it." I flew home the following day, somehow knowing they wouldn't follow-up. Six months later, the girl suffered a large hemorrhage which left her partially paralyzed. To my knowledge, she's still living with her AVM.

I brought home some lessons from my trips to Colombia that may have relevance to our own health care system, to the way we train our doctors and perhaps most importantly to what a visiting "expert" can offer to a struggling surgical environment. It's hard to experience up close the deep discrepancies in the availability and quality of neurosurgical care in a third-world country without reflecting on health care as a basic human right as opposed to a privilege reserved for the political / economic elite. In the same fashion one can't help but recognize that what a country like Columbia needs is emphatically not more high-tech neurosurgeons driving Land Cruisers but rather a tightly-woven, pyramidal-shaped medical infrastructure with the means for early diagnosis and acute referral to a limited number of centralized well-equipped surgical specialty units where a few guys like Roberto, our flap-turner, and Dr. Joaquin Rodriguez could provide superb service to a high volume of patients.

Finally, I think the contrast between my two AVM cases- the one I 'did" with Joaquin Rodriquez and the one I bailed on with Dr. Segovia- points up the proper role of the visiting fireman. Dr. Joaquin has gone on to become an important go-to guy in Columbian neurosurgery; he'd have done that without my minor input but I flatter myself by believing he's a little better AVM surgeon as a result of our shared experience. On the other hand, my ignoring the obvious difficulty of the second AVM, and then -for a variety of pitiable reasons- electing to proceed without the appropriate prerequisites in planning, assistance, equipment, and anesthesia is not only terrible patient care but equally importantly, sets exactly the wrong example for anyone who cares to look.

CHAPTER SEVENTEEN

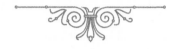

Patients

T
he previous pages contain a lot of information about people as patients, folks I've encountered in the management of specific diseases or in unique circumstances, meaning that more often than not, the patient him or herself has not been the real focus of my story. I want to change now to write briefly about five very special patients as people -individuals whose personalities have made indelible marks on my life and my career. They've all graciously agreed to me telling their stories.

GINA WILSON

A young woman I'll call Gina was in her mid-twenties when first we met. Gina was a sweet, pleasant East Texas girl working in her small town's library when out of nowhere she suffered a seizure. Seizures come in several flavors; Gina's was the full monte, what medicine calls a Grand Mal fit, complete with the sudden onset of unconsciousness, drawing up of arms and legs followed by uncontrollable shaking and finally a limp state of coma. During the several minute process the patient falls down, may bite her lip or tongue and generally loses control of her bladder; consequently, she wakes up on the floor surrounded by horrified onlookers, lying in a pool of urine and blood with no idea what's happened. Pretty disconcerting at the local library.

After an initial work-up Gina was sent over to see me because her imaging studies had demonstrated a large non-dominant hemisphere arterio-venous malformation without evidence of bleeding. Seizures are the presenting symptoms in some one-third of AVM patients, and generally can be successfully treated using medication without removing the malformation. The larger risk that every AVM portends is an ultimate hemorrhage, so once the diagnosis has been made in the evaluation of the seizure, attention turns to what should /can be done about the AVM itself.

The hemorrhage risk of an unruptured AVM has been the subject of great debate in Neurology and Neurosurgery for over fifty years; recently it's been more or less pinned down at roughly 2.2 % annually, with a mortality rate of each bleed of 10% and a serious morbidity of around 20%. That translates as "If you have an AVM and live long enough, odds are it's going to bleed, and when it does there's a I out of 3 chance you'll die or be badly hurt". Another way to calculate the lifetime risk of bleeding is to subtract the patient's age from 108; for Gina, that meant she had about a 4 out of 5 chance of hemorrhaging in her anticipated life span.

Those are daunting numbers for a twenty-six-year-old, but they have to be compared with the potential risks and complications of treatment, which in the late 1970s were enormous. Gina's malformation was too large to be treated successfully in any way but by surgery. The AVM was located in and around portions of the brain responsible for most of the motor function in her left face, arm and leg. Surgical removal would unquestionably leave her weak to paralyzed on the left side of her body; in addition, even successful resection had less than a 50-50 chance to cure her seizures. More importantly, such an operation carried a risk to her life (during or immediately after the procedure) of 15-20%. A no-brainer, as we say.

Faced with a situation like this, I've learned from my friend Roberto Heros, an outstanding AVM surgeon, to emphasize the "good news" in the following fashion:

"Gina, let's look at it this way. The AVM may never hemorrhage, and in fact, if it does some time in the future, there's a two out of three chance that you'll live through it and be pretty normal afterwards. Plus, if a hemorrhage does happen, by that time, our treatment options will definitely be better than they are currently. I'll watch you closely, and if anything changes, we'll re-evaluate the situation then." Far easier for me to say than for her to live with, but it was all we had.

Gina was started on anti-seizure medication and for almost six months was fine. Then she had a small bleed from the AVM which transiently left her with a very weak left leg. She recovered almost completely over about a month, during which time she decided she just couldn't live with the uncertainty of the AVM for the remainder of her life. Unwilling to bite the bullet, I sent her to see some of my slick neurosurgery colleagues around the country, but everybody said the risk of removing the AVM was too great, so Gina came back to Texas and had two more small bleeds over a period of six months.

After her third hemorrhage, she recovered well neurologically but emotionally Gina was a wreck, as were her parents. I saw her for a protracted clinic visit once every other week, and was close to becoming a wreck myself, which didn't change my awareness that, on my best day, I couldn't remove that malformation without either ruining or even killing her.

At this time, I was fresh out of the Army where I'd spent my final year at its flagship hospital in Washington D.C. One day of each week there, I'd go down to the lab to operate some rats and fool around with whatever nutty experiments were going on. One of these, being done by a friend, focused on trying to glue tissue together, especially traumatized soft tissue, as in battlefield wounds. A part of the project looked at joining ruptured blood vessels together, especially tiny ones like those I 'd learned to sew together in YSG's lab in Zurich. My buddy wasn't having much luck, because the several types of cyanoacrylate adhesives ("crazy glue") available all seemed one hell of a lot better at plugging the vessels up rather than keeping them open.

We injected the stuff in some rat aortas and found that even small amounts of the glue would fill the entire downstream circulation almost before we could remove the injection needle, simply because the adhesive polymerized so rapidly. That would definitely be a problem if we planned to use it in people, but at least superficially the concept seemed to have some potential in the treatment of AVMs. Since there are no animal models of AVMs, we were stumped for a next move, and just about that time my service commitment was up and I hustled back to Texas.

It took a while back home to get any kind of a lab set up, and I was still more interested in sewing things together as opposed to injecting crazy glue, but just before I met Gina, I'd begun fooling around with various types and mixtures of cyanoacrylate, again in rats and in some rabbits after they'd been used for other experiments. The stuff was very effective in blocking off arteries and veins on direct injection, but it polymerized so rapidly that most of the time it didn't even reach the smaller vessels, and it was tricky to use, with the injection needle bonding immediately to everything it touched.

When some early reports came out of Europe suggesting the polymerization time could be extended and the injectate made radiographically visible by mixing in a dye normally used for myelography, I thought that sounded promising, so I investigated the mixture in a variety of animal arteries. The results were imprecise, but in fact, by varying the concentration of the glue, I could delay the polymerization time somewhat and any X-Rays I could manage to arrange after injection did show traces of the IBCA in the occluded vessels.

So, after talking to Gina, I contacted the FDA, explained the clinical situation and ultimately received a "compassionate drug exemption", meaning that, if there were no other options, I had permission to use the IBCA in this one patient. There was a fair amount of paper work for both of us to complete, during which time we continued to discuss the possibilities. I figured that at the best, blocking off some of the malformation with IBCA would reduce the risk of her bleeding to death during an operation and might slightly diminish any damage I'd do to the surrounding brain, but I wasn't kidding her or myself about the probable long-term result; at best, she'd be crippled on her left side.

"But if the AVM is gone, I won't be worrying about another stroke and bleeding to death, right?" I said, "Probably," because really I didn't know.

Finally, following another small bleed, I set Gina up for surgery. My plan was to expose the major arteries going to the AVM, inject each with a slug of crazy glue, then to do an angiogram on the operating table to see how much AVM was left. If the angio results suggested I could successfully remove the residual malformation, I'd proceed with surgery; if not, then I'd do some more injections.

Since, as far as I was aware, this hadn't been done in a human being (and as I said,there were no animal models) I was pretty much winging it, and Gina was along for the ride. We spent hours in my office talking about the process.

The night prior to operation, again I went through every possibility I could imagine and how I planned to handle each one. She asked good questions and a lot of them. For most, I just didn't have any answers, other than I'd try to get the AVM out and keep her alive while doing it. Gina said, "I believe you", and signed her op permit.

The following morning everything went according to plan. We isolated three of the larger arteries which supplied her AVM and I carefully injected each one with a mixture of the dye and the glue. The sole hitch came on the final injection, when either the mixture was wrong or, more likely, I delayed a second or so longer than I should have before withdrawing the injection needle. The damn thing stuck in the artery, and it was never coming out.

Even this wasn't terrible news. This particular artery was located deep in the seam between the two frontal lobes about 2 ½ inches below the surface of the brain ; the needle itself was three inches long and when I detached it from the injection syringe, its hub was barely visible at the level of the cortex, and the shaft lay up against the fibrous septum (falx) that separates the two hemispheres. There are no moving parts within the skull, so once I knew I couldn't get the needle out without tearing the artery, I just sutured it to the septum and figured we'd dodged a real bullet. That was right before we did the angiogram.

The study showed one good thing. It appeared that there was a lot less blood going through the AVM now. Everything else was bad news. Rather than amputating or blocking off a large segment of the malformation, thus making it simpler to remove, the glue had simply hollowed the malformation out, decreasing the blood flow to areas near the center of the AVM, but leaving the periphery untouched . Even worse, those small parts of the AVM that I could actually see on the brain's surface were filled with threads of stiff, brittle glue. Now, rather than being soft and pliable, the malformation was like a mottled sea urchin buried in brain tissue. There was no way to remove it without taking out all the adjacent brain, most of which was still working. So, I closed Gina's head. When she emerged from the anesthetic, she was much weaker in both her arm and leg, but I'd prepared her for that.

What neither of us were prepared for was the uncertain future. What did this new creature I'd created in her brain mean going forward? Would it cause the rest of the AVM to progressively clot off? Would the change in flow pattern make a hemorrhage more likely, less likely? What would happen with her seizures (which came from the brain around the AVM, not the AVM itself)? Crying, Gina asked me, "How can you not know?"

But I didn't. And as far as I could determine, neither did anyone else anywhere in the neurosurgical world. So, I recommended we wait it out while she recovered from the initial operation, which took almost six months. Meanwhile I repeated her angiogram twice; there was no appreciable change in the size or flow dynamics of the AVM on either study. During that time, Gina had no more seizure activity and I kept my fingers crossed, hoping that meant something good was going on that we just couldn't see.

Thirteen months after her surgery Gina had a fourth small hemorrhage from her AVM, followed two days later by a bigger bleed which left her almost completely paralyzed on her left side. This made a total of five hemorrhages since her diagnosis. I didn't know what role the glue injection played in the last two, but there was no evidence it had made things better. A week after her last bleed, I took the AVM out, glue and all, in about eight bloody hours, and then I followed Gina for 24 years. She never had another hemorrhage, for which she was grateful, but she remained densely hemi-plegic. The last time I saw her she told me, "Living like this is hell."

JUDY PRATER

I believe there are different types of courage, but learning - as a teenager - that you have an incurable brain disease and then squeezing a "normal life" out of the consequences requires a special vintage of bravery almost beyond comprehension. Judy was a teenager when we first met. She'd had a grand mal seizure at school in San Antonio, and after recovering completely in about six hours was found to have a giant AVM that involved her dominant left frontal and temporal lobes, extending deep into the basal ganglia and down into the ventricular system of that hemisphere. This monster measured about 7 cm x 6 cm x 5 cm and had arterial feeding from almost of the brain's arteries, several of which were studded with aneurysms, blister-like weaknesses produced by the abnormally high blood flow, each aneurysm representing its own risk of catastrophic bleeding. Despite all this, Judy was an almost normal teenager, with only a slight trace of weakness in her right face and right upper extremity. She was bright, pleasant and engaged. Not only that, she had perhaps the most supportive family I would ever encounter.

Judy hadn't had a hemorrhage yet, but it wasn't long in coming, a mild one that kept her in hospital for with a bad headache and some speech disturbance for several days. We repeated her angiogram; nothing had changed with the AVM and I had exactly nothing to offer her. I thought, with enough blood transfusions, I could probably take this thing out, but knew for certain I would leave her hemi-plegic, completely aphasic and blind in at least one-half of her visual fields. And with an AVM, there are no partial measures- not then and not now. Anything done to the malformation that doesn't completely remove it has no effect on the risk of further bleeding, other than perhaps actually increasing that possibility. So, we did nothing but watch.

Over the ensuing two decades Judy graduated from college, married Jon Prater and had two children. She and her husband moved with his employment around the US, and at about every stop, Judy would have another bleed. Each hemorrhage would take a small permanent bite out of her neurological function, and almost always she'd undergo another angiogram in hopes that somehow something would have changed that would make the AVM treatable. No such luck. In the process she was evaluated by the best AVM surgeons in the country. I'd get a telephone call from a friend in Phoenix, San Francisco, Miami or New York, all saying 'we only wish we could think of some way to help'. Judy kept right on living and loving and coping with her gradually increasing disability.

By the time Judy and her family made their way back to Texas, the train was coming off the tracks. She'd had five hemorrhages- the mortality rate with each bleed is around 10%- so the odds were slipping away from her. Even worse, she was steadily losing function in her right arm and leg, and her speech was deteriorating. These losses were not all the result of hemorrhages. Some were caused by a wicked, paradoxical phenomena called "cerebral steal", in which, since the AVM has very low resistance in its vessels because of the lack of any capillary system, arterial blood is almost sucked into the malformation and away from normal brain tissue. This "steal" produces ischemia, or a paucity of blood flow, in normal brain tissue, and when the "steal" is profound and prolonged, as in Julie's case, the normal brain cells first stutter like a car running out of gas, then cease working and finally actually infarct or die. Judy was experiencing actual "strokes' from lack of blood flow in the normal brain adjacent to her AVM, in addition to her repetitive hemorrhages.

Judy never came to my clinic without her family; almost always her husband, usually her mother, frequently her father and often her young children. The only time I ever saw her cry was when, after all these hemorrhages, I explained the slow, unfair "steal" process that was crippling her. She looked at her husband and mother and very carefully said, "I can't live like this." Then, to me, "Please help me." We were all crying then. I asked for a couple of weeks to think things over again and sent her home.

I had a new partner then, a young man named Guy West. This joker had come to spend three years with us learning to treat vascular diseases after completion of his residency in Washington. Despite being a fan of the despicable Redskins, he proved to be just too good to let get away, so we kept him around on the faculty for comic relief if nothing else. He'd seen Judy with me a couple of times, and after her most recent visit I asked him to help me design a plan of attack that would address the "steal' problem and maybe, just maybe, reduce the possibility of her having more hemorrhages. After some preliminary discussion we recruited our expert in focused radiation therapy, Tommy Whitson, and over a period of about three weeks came up with something that sounded like it might possibly work.

Focused radiation therapy has been shown to be effective in obliterating AVMs but it generally requires up to two years to be effective, and, because of its deleterious effects on surrounding brain is really useful only in smaller malformations. Tommy decided to programmatically divide Judy's AVM up into small portions, each of which would be irradiated at different intervals. If the radiation actually was effective, as scar tissue formed in the AVM, there would be more resistance to the blood passing through it, resistance which would increase the pressure inside the arteries, making a hemorrhage from one of her multiple aneurysms more likely, so we would need to deal with those aneurysms on the front end of our treatment plan.

Guy, trained in both open microsurgery and endo-vascular surgery (meaning using a catheter), felt pretty sure he could eliminate all of the aneurysms in a couple of sittings. Once we got that far, after radiation and aneurysm treatment, the next step would be to isolate the blood supply to the AVM, basically disconnecting the arteries going to the malformation from those supplying normal brain. That would require at least one and maybe two open operative procedures. To complete the entire treatment plan would require at least 24 months.

To list all the potential complications of this type protocol would require multiple pages of fine print, but in two long clinic visits with Judy and her family the three of us – Guy, Tommy and the old man- did as complete a job as possible. The major risks were straight-forward: we could hurt her directly with the embolization, the surgery and or the radiation, the operation(s) or the embolization could cause the AVM or the aneurysms to hemorrhage, we could injure critical arteries going to normal brain or, more likely, the procedures might go well but the whole plan might fail. The alternative was to do nothing, and Judy wanted no part of that. From her wheelchair she gave me a big hug, a crooked smile and a halting "Thank you." Judy Prater was a truly courageous young woman.

It was a good plan; I'd try it again. Tommy did some creative stuff with the Gamma Knife in several sittings, while Guy took care of the aneurysms and did a masterful job disconnecting normal from abnormal vessels. Over the first nine months of treatment Judy seemed to stabilize and perhaps, although this may have been just my wishful thinking, even improve a little with respect to her speech. Her angiogram and MRI both looked as if we were making progress because there was a marked reduction in the blood flow through the AVM, and Guy and I remarked that at least from a technical point of view, we could theoretically take the damn thing out at this point. Everyone, especially Judy's family, was optimistic. If we could just hold what we had while the radiation effects shriveled up more of the AVM, there was a reasonable chance Judy would come through this minimally worse for the experience.

Unfortunately, the AVM always gets a vote. Almost one year after starting treatment Judy Prater suffered a massive hemorrhage. Guy saved her life by emergently removing the remnants of the AVM and the huge clot, but she was neurologically devastated. She has subsequently undergone several more operations, but requires continual care; her husband, children and devoted parents are with her as often as is possible . Despite recognizing them, her ability to interact with her loved ones is limited.

LEM MOLSON

When I came out of the service to start my practice in 1977, in Texas at least there was still a significant residual antipathy between the "hippies" and the "straights", even though the hippy community was being, believe it or not, rapidly absorbed into the urban redneck mainstream of Janis Joplin, Willie Nelson etc. Since even hippies have to eat, lots of folks on that edge of the American social fabric found jobs in government service, more specifically in the US Post Office. Granted, you had to wear a uniform – Bermuda shorts and a short-sleeved shirt in Texas- but no one told you how long your hair, beard or mustache had to be, what and where your tats were and whether you could wear jewelry in your nose, lips, ears or eyebrows. The work itself was steady but not too tiresome, you met a variety of folks and to top it all off, you could wear a pith helmet in the summer. Add in a steady paycheck and it was hard to beat.

I know all this because of a young man named Lem Molson, a 28-year-old postal "carrier" who was under my care for about three months that first summer I was back in Texas. At a casual glance we weren't much of a match; I was freshly discharged from the Army, proud of my service and, except for a nascent beard, looked it. Lem was short and skinny, with long hair worn in a grubby ponytail, ear ring, nose ring and lip ring, with every visible centimeter of skin covered with ink artistry. He'd been a conscientious objector throughout the Vietnam War during which he'd gone to Canada for a while with the thought of immigrating. Unfortunately, he couldn't stand the winters and didn't like their brand of country music, so he made his way back to Texas in 1973. Lem marched in every protest march he could find in North Texas (not heavy work) and mostly was against things.

About the only subject Lem was radically on board with was marriage, and that was solely because he was deeply in love with Rhonda, his wife of two years. Rhonda, a stringy blond woman a couple years older than Lem, worked in a Legal Aid office and thought her husband was 'the neatest thing since Mexican Marijuana'. I know because that's the way she described him the day the two of them showed up in my clinic, begging me to save their marriage.

Their problem was sex. Here were two healthy, horny young people who barely could keep their hands off one another in my office, both scared out of their minds to have intercourse because of Lem's headaches. To make a tearful long story short, Rhonda and Lem both really liked sex, and a lot of it (at age 37 just listening to them made me tired). The problem was that in the last three months almost every time Lem got "lathered up"- Rhonda's description- he suddenly developed a "killer of a headache" that often wouldn't disappear for days. The last episode had been so terrible he went to a local ER where the docs couldn't find anything specifically wrong. His routine x-rays were normal (CT scans weren't routinely available in North Texas until 1978) and they'd even done a spinal tap that showed just a tinge of blood in Lem's spinal fluid; the ER felt probably this was what we call a traumatic tap, meaning a small blood vessel in Lem's dura had been nicked by the needle.

Despite lack of evidence, Lem's misery was so convincing that he was admitted to hospital. The following day a local neurosurgeon had done an arteriogram, which he and the attending radiologist agreed, was "stone cold normal". Lem was discharged with a prescription for Valium and a referral to a young psychologist, Paul Chesser, who happened to be my weekend racquetball partner.

Following Lem's initial psychological session, the not-so-mild-mannered shrink called me. "Professor, one of your medical bozos has royally screwed the pooch here. Both these kids are crying like babies in my office; their life is sweeter than any two kids their age deserve, and all they want to do is screw one another. They've even given up pot, because both are afraid he's going die every time he gets an erection. This young man is terribly depressed but it ain't because his id is dissing his ego. I want you to take a look, and I'll spot your lame ass two points every game on Saturday."

He was lying about the two points, but this was my kind of referral, so I saw Lem and Rhonda the next day. I've always hated being late to clinic- it's impolite and demeaning to patients- but sometimes you just get stuck, and often when that happens patients are extremely and understandably pissed. These two had been waiting over an hour when I went out in the waiting room with a big apology that never got past my lips. You would have thought I was Jimmi Hendrix re-incarnated the way those kids jumped up, both saying "thanks you so much for seeing me/him." I felt even worse when Rhonda grabbed my arm and almost moaned, "Please believe us Doctor Samson."

Well, as far as I could tell, Lem was normal. His neck might have been a little stiff for a skinny guy, but he's been sleeping on the sofa for weeks to avoid any of those semi-conscious amorous encounters I could recall with fondness. His x-rays, to include an arteriogram that appeared to have been done by a rank amateur, at first glance failed to provide any clues. Brad, the resident who was helping with the exam that afternoon was truly worthless (we ultimately cut him loose about a year later) so when he squealed and pointed at the top of the sheet of x-ray film, I was not impressed.

"Look, Boss, they cut off the top of his skull." No shit; the lateral x-ray tube had been so mal-positioned that about two inches of the top of the brain to include the vessels therein, were missing. I know in my heart I would have noticed if I'd kept looking.

About 85% of all aneurysms occur right at the base of the brain, where the four major arteries come together in what's known as the Circle of Willis. The remaining fifteen percent are located out on the periphery; when we finally re-did Lem's angiogram that's where his was, stuck out on the ass-end of a small artery known as the callosal marginal. It's a pretty easy surgical fix, and when I exposed it that same afternoon, the surrounding brain was stained with the remnants of several prior hemorrhages. Lem was in the hospital for about four days. When I sent him home, I gave both of them the surgical stink-eye and said I wanted him to "take it easy" for a couple of weeks.

Before the cell phone era, we all carried "beepers", infernal devices that screeched a mechanical tune and displayed a telephone number, usually that of our answering service. Late that evening the number was one I didn't know, with a Fort Worth area code. Like a zombie, I found a pay telephone and fifty cents; Rhoda's squeaky voice answered on the first ring.

"The trifecta, Dr. Duke! The trifecta- what did you do to him?" All things considered, she sounded pretty happy.

PAUL BEST

I mistakenly married an aspiring socialite in 1982, and immediately was exposed to a social circle I'd had no clue existed previously. Politicians, wheelers, dealers, models, hangers-on and a few really nice folks- none of whom I would have come to know in the routine order of things. Soon thereafter, at one of what seemed to be an endless succession of cocktail parties, I was introduced to Paul Best, a local "investments guy", bon vivant and man about town. Paul was about 10 years my senior, had grown up poor in East Texas, worked like a dog on the family farm before scraping through a small college and then coming to the big city to make his fortune.

Paul was what's been described as a "people person". When I met him, he was holding court and telling stories to a circle of other beautiful people, cigarette in one hand and a large Martini in the other. When my new wife introduced us, he promptly handed off both the drink and the smoke so he could give me the grip and a big hug simultaneously. I disliked the son-of-a-bitch on first sight.

It turned out Paul was the front man for his investment firm and ran his life right at the red line most of the time. He was short, overweight, sweaty and kind of all over you in every encounter; he smoked like a chimney, drank copious amounts, played lots of terrible golf and knew more gossip about the "people that counted" in finance and politics than arguably anybody in Texas. He also was a shrewd interpreter of unspoken conversations, later telling my wife in private that "I don't think the big guy likes me very much."

She assured him I was just "sorta anti-social and slow to warm up to new friends." They were both right.

The more I heard about Paul Best the more it became obvious he was a great businessman, a real cheerleader for the city and a force to be reckoned with in the affluent society that got things done in the big town. Privately, it looked like to me Paul was going to have a pretty brief run because his health was on a short fuse. The number of medications he took was a frequent topic of his own jocular conversation, and other than golf, his favorite form of exercise was rattling the Martini shaker. As he told me once later, at that point in his life his major goal in life was to die full and out of debt. Ironically, he was married to one of the sweetest woman I'd ever met, but Paul and I didn't have much in common, so I found it easy to have previous obligations when we were invited socially by the Bests.

Late night–early morning ER calls are often water-marks in neurosurgeon's lives. At midnight on a summer evening, when my boss, the chief of surgery, called to tell me Paul Best was in our ER with "my kind of stroke", I climbed in my truck with a premonition of badness. Sure enough, after fighting my way through the cluster of society stars in the ER waiting area, I found Paul and his wife Karla in one of the Trauma Rooms where he'd just returned from angiography. He was almost aphasic with a right facial weakness and a weak right upper extremity; classical presentation of a left middle cerebral artery stroke, except for the fact his right lower extremity was also weak. There wasn't much call for sophisticated neurological diagnosis, because he'd already had the definitive test, an arteriogram of his brain circulation which demonstrated complete occlusion of his left internal carotid artery high in his neck.

For technical reasons, this kind of blockage couldn't be treated directly in 1983, especially not in the middle of the night. If the lack of blood supply persisted for several more hours, Paul's brain tissue, some of which was stuttering along now, would be irreversibly damaged, so the clock was literally ticking. There was one slim surgical option, invented by my old mentor Professor Yasargil, an option which played to mixed reviews in terms of its efficacy. This procedure involved using a small artery in the scalp as a so-called "brain bypass", surgically joining it to a branch of the ischemic middle cerebral artery on the brain's surface. The operation is a little more complex than I've made it sound; first the surgeon has to dissect the scalp artery free, then drill a hole in the skull over the area of the recipient vessel and finally sew both arteries, which are about the size of a number 2 pencil lead, together with suture the diameter of human hair. But it was doable, and for better or worse, both in rats and people, I'd done a bunch.

So, I gave Paul and Karla an abbreviated version of the possibilities (treat with aspirin, fluids, anti-swelling medications and hope... or do this, right now), the potentials (operation might work, might not, might make you worse, you might die) and the promise (we'll take the best care of you possible, whatever you decide).

Karla cried, but Paul looked at me and nodded his head. All he could say was" bubba". So we went to the OR. As far as Paul and I were concerned, for the rest of his life, I was "Bubba."

The surgery went well; the procedure itself isn't difficult, just tedious. Before closing, we did a quick angiogram to prove the bypass was open – I was gratefully surprised at how much blood was pumping into the ischemic area. Paul woke up just the same neurologically as he was before the operation. By the next morning his speech was better but not fluent and his CT scan showed us a small permanent infarct in his left frontal lobe. He left the hospital at nine days post-op almost but not quite neurologically normal and lived another 22 years until multiple cardiac infarcts destroyed his heart. It's those 22 years that make this brief story important.

Neither Paul nor I ever knew if the bypass made a difference. He was convinced it did, and I was skeptical, but there wasn't then and isn't now definitive information about "re-vascularization" in the acute setting of a stroke (his bypass was completed within 5 hours of the onset of his symptoms). And, as he reminded me more than once, "Bubba, we were out of options, and you sure as hell didn't make me any worse." What the entire experience did do was to make him different.

When Paul came back to work, he didn't stop smoking or drinking, although he honestly tried, and intermittently made a little progress. He didn't stop going to parties or giving speeches or making money, but what he did do was focus all of his amazing energies on making health care better, more comprehensive and more accessible, especially for folks without money. He'd been involved before with Metropolitan, our city-county hospital, but now he became immersed in every aspect of its development, as long as that development translated directly into better care for more people. Tirelessly he served on every board, committee and taskforce we could come up with, His only demand was that the goal or target wasn't decorative or administrative or anything except making the care of individuals safer, more effective and more available. He didn't try to impersonate a doctor, but he asked hard, penetrating questions about every proposal that crossed his desk. More than one self-important physician slunk away from Paul's come-to-Jesus budgetary sessions wishing he'd never tried to sneak some bullshit proposal wrapped in medical jargon past that chunky guy with the scar on his head at the end of the table.

Paul and Karla were two of my few former patients that grew into close friends. When I finally came to my senses and dumped my would-be-socialite, I figured they'd be one of the few things we'd accumulated together that I would miss. I gave the two of them a lot of slack, but that never happened; Paul made a point of showing up at my office unannounced one afternoon to say, "Bubba, me and Karla are in this with you for the long haul."

And that's the way it turned out. For the next two decades, they were both there for Patricia, our sons and me, every time and all the time.

Paul died in April at the end of a long ICU convalescence following a "Hail Mary" heart operation from which he just couldn't recover. He and Karla had introduced our family to Northwest Montana, and it was his fervent wish through all that miserable winter just to make it back to the Flathead Valley one more time. Sitting at his bedside right before Patricia and I left for a three-day spring vacation, I made certain he knew breakfast was on me the next time we ate at the Echo Lake Café up in Bigfork. It was evening and he was too tired to really talk, so he just said "Miss you, Bubba." Or maybe it was, "I'll miss you, Bubba."

Paul Best's massive heart failed for the last time on the second day of our trip. Karla took his ashes back to Northwest Montana that summer.

MARLENE DECKER

The human brain is encased in the densest bone of the skeletal system. Evolution designed things that way because the brain is almost pathetically easy to injure. Roughly the consistency of Jello left out of the refrigerator overnight, you can cut the brain with a dull spoon or bruise it with the thump of a careless finger. Its blood vessels bleed like stink because they're so fragile, and there's no surrounding tissue to tamponade the hemorrhage. Protracted bleeding stimulates the arteries to spasm, which can produce a stroke, and only a small amount of free blood will foul up the spinal fluid absorption system, resulting in permanent hydrocephalus. The nerve cells themselves (neurons) die when injured and never regenerate; their scar tissue can make adjacent neurons ignite randomly, resulting in any one of several types of seizures. It's a wonder anyone lives after brain trauma, especially anyone older than 15.

Marlene Decker, by all accounts a lovely 57-year-old lady, was jogging in her suburban neighborhood on a Saturday morning when a second nice lady blew through a stop sign, launching Mrs. Decker through the air to a hard landing on the pavement. Within twenty minutes, she was in the Metropolitan Memorial Hospital Emergency Room with a Glasgow Coma Score of 5 and a fixed, dilated right pupil. Coma scores range from 16 (normal) to 3 (present and breathing); a fixed and dilated pupil in the absence of eye or orbital injury indicates a large mass (usually a clot) compressing the brain on that side.

My partner, Guy West, was in the hospital making rounds when he was called to the ER by our residents to evaluate this lady. Her skull films showed a large fracture; given her deteriorating condition, without further ado, Dr. West whipped Marlene upstairs and removed roughly half of her skull. This operation, called a hemi-craniectomy, was devised in the late 1960s to treat massive brain trauma because the life- threatening aspects of these injuries are of two types. The most immediate risks are blood clots, developing either over the brain surface or in its battered and bruised tissues; these represent acute threats to survival because of their pressure on the brain stem. The second type threat -the swelling or edema produced by the injury- is a relentless process which generally becomes maximum at 48-72 hours post-injury and kills just as effectively as an immediate hematoma.

To address these dual threats, a hemi-craniectomy surgically removes almost all of the bone overlaying one half of the cortex, an area roughly described by a line extending from in front of the ear to the outside of the orbit, then to the midline of the forehead; from that point, the removal proceeds posteriorly in the mid-line, all the way back to the bony "knob" of the occiput and finally back to the ear. The total amount of skull removed is about the size of a man's hand with the fingers wide-spread; this so-called 'bone flap" is subsequently frozen in a sterile container, hopefully to be replaced at a later date. Some hemi-craniectomies remove bone above the forehead on both sides of the mid-line, but the unilateral hemi-craniectomy I've described above is by far the most common.

The outer covering of the brain- the dura mater- is located just below the skull. Clots secondary to trauma can form either superficial or deep to this membrane, which when intact, restricts any brain expansion due to swelling or post-injury edema. Thus, when dealing with almost all serious traumatic brain injuries, the hemi-craniectomy is combined with a wide opening of the dura, an opening which may or may not be closed with a graft of some type, according to the circumstances, the surgeon's preferences, the phase of the moon, etc.

Dr. West did all this and a little more, removing a huge clot in the space below the dura in addition to a small amount of traumatized frontal lobe that was certain to be a problem later, then he closed Mrs. D's scalp loosely over a drain left in the epidural space. Skin-to-skin, he was in and out in a little over two hours -rocket speed- then Mrs. Decker went straight for what would be her first CT scan. Guy knew she wasn't out of the woods when the scan showed extensive bruising of both the right frontal and temporal poles, which are the tips of those lobes situated immediately beneath the skull itself. In addition, there was some ominous, early generalized brain edema. He told Robert, Marlene's husband, that the next several days would be touch and go. Depending on your definition of "several", Guy was correct.

Over the next week and a half Marlene went back to the OR twice, both times for further "decompression", removal of damaged brain tissue that had "blossomed" into large confluent hemorrhages which themselves produced dramatic, intolerable increases in brain volume. Her neurological condition waxed and waned from bad to poor as the ICU team pulled out all the stops to keep her intra-cranial pressure consistent with life. She had one piece of luck; her brain's damaged hemisphere was the right one, the so-called non-dominant hemisphere, meaning the side opposite her centers of language function. This laterality was one of the major reasons Guy and his team fought doggedly to keep her alive through every imaginable complication. If they could just get her "over this hump", Marlene had a chance to be most of a functional human being again.

This "hump" was pretty steep. After her three decompressive craniotomies, Marlene developed hydrocephalus, the inability to re-absorb her spinal fluid, and required a shunting procedure to divert the fluid from her brain into her abdominal cavity, Then, just as it appeared there was some light at the end of the tunnel, her entire scalp flap – the huge amount of skin that covered her hemi-craniectomy defect – turned black and died. This complication was probably an effect of the skin having been reflected back on itself multiple times for protracted time periods and perhaps evidence that we weren't padding it sufficiently during one or more of the operations.

To address this complication, we enlisted the help of Jim Thorton, a fantastic plastic surgeon, who designed and then harvested a full thickness skin flap from Marlene's chest wall to cover the giant defect. He returned her to the OR after the flap had "matured" to help us replace the bone flap Guy had removed and to re-make the skull. Jim also neatened up the soft tissue around the edges of our lengthy incision, the kind of little thing brain surgeons think is insignificant, but patients and families do not.

I helped Guy take care of Marlene and Robert during the latter part of her four-month long ICU stay, then with him followed her as an out-patient over the ensuing nine years. This length of follow-up is unusual for a neurosurgical patient relationship. Frankly, almost all our patients injured this badly die during the initial stages of their illnesses, while those less seriously hurt leave our surveillance when their neurological status stabilizes. Serendipitously, the protracted length and sustained intensity of our follow-up provided all of her care-givers a degree of insight to Marlene's recovery that was startling.

For starters, this fortunate lady had a tremendous amount of family support. Her husband and children were as dedicated as was humanly possible and her family had sufficient resources to insure the consistent kind of support you'd wish for every brain-injured patient. However, completely separate and apart from that, Marlene proved to be simply one of the toughest, most determined patients any of us had ever seen. Everyday, she worked her ass off to get better, and slowly, painfully, almost incrementally, over months and then years, she did just that.

As a general rule of thumb, somewhere around 9-12 months after the adult brain has been injured, what you see is what the patient is going to have to live with. Not this time- at one-year post-injury, Marlene was just getting warmed up.

Walking, talking, reading, remembering, using her hand; step by painful step she learned to do it all, with a stubborn gracefulness that took all of her care-givers' breath away. There were some hitches on the road- some "minor" procedures requiring hospitalization which were important; she hated each and every one, I think because they represented set-backs to her goal of being well and perhaps sub-conscious threats to her hard-won independence. During each one, we couldn't keep her in the hospital one minute beyond the absolute minimum. Following one such accelerated discharge, she refused to visit me as an out-patient because our last two encounters had resulted in hospitalization.

Like many physicians, I'm a skeptic about "willing" oneself to be healthy. If the brain ain't working, you can "will" all you want but that arm or leg just won't move. But Marlene is living, breathing proof that if you want to badly enough, a few thousand reluctant neurons can be compelled do the work of a million dead ones. This courageous lady is not neurologically normal, but by virtue of sheer grit, Marlene Decker is an independent, functional, admirable woman. She's become my definition of indomitable, and it's been an enduring pleasure to have played a minor role in her care. Just another reason why, from start to stop, this has been the best job in the world.

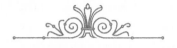

CHAPTER EIGHTEEN

Teaching

Our chief resident in 1985 at the time of the Delta 1011 crash was a young man named Tim Lord. He'd grown up in a large South Texas city where his father had been the first trained neurosurgeon between Houston and Dallas. Tom was smart, hardnosed and straight as an arrow; while playing football at SMU he may have once thought about something other than neurosurgery as a career, but by the time we got him for residency training he was locked on like a heat-seeking missile. After he dazzled everybody in his first two years, I started hatching a plot to keep him on our faculty when he finished. I dangled that possibility the next autumn over drinks at a meeting in San Francisco, telling him how, with his help, we would conquer American Neurosurgery and he'd become internationally famous, but he wasn't having any of it.

"Boss, I really appreciate your confidence in me, but once you hand me that diploma, I'm going back home. I'm joining my dad's old group if they'll have me, then we'll see if I can make a living as a simple country brain surgeon."

"Tim, I may have been born at night, but it wasn't last night. That 'aw shucks" bullshit just won't cut it.

You've got a ton of talent, you're really good with people, you never even thought a lie and you're one of the hardest working residents I've seen. So, whatever you decide to do and wherever you want to do it, we both know you're going to be an instant success. I'm just asking you to give some thought to using those gifts here with us- building this clinical program, teaching residents how to become real neurosurgeons, and maybe focusing on brain tumors or something else to get a national reputation. Plus, I just like having your sorry ass around."

We both laughed, and he said, "Well, I'll think about it." Only he sounded like he probably wouldn't.

I let the offer slide for the moment. One of the nice things about neurosurgery training programs is their small size. At that moment we had two residents at each level of a five-year program and six total faculty surgeons, so everyone was interacting with everyone else on a routine basis for a protracted time. That, added to the intensity of the disease states we treated, made for a highly pressurized, almost intimate working environment. I knew I'd be seeing Tim up close and personal on an almost daily basis for the next two years.

The topic raised its ugly head a final time about six months later during one of our quarterly resident evaluation sessions. Tim and our other chief resident were sitting in and contributing to a no-holds-barred discussion that for the moment was centered on the sub-par performance of one of our second- year trainees. "Smiley" Riley, the young man in question, didn't seem to have a clue how to do his job, and worse, didn't actually seem to give a damn, despite prior extensive counselling. We were on the brink of placing him on probation, and today the specific issue under consideration was Riley's operative skills- or lack thereof. The chief prosecutor was one of our tumor surgeons, a Brazilian-born slick surgical technician I'll Dr. Tano.

"Theese guy can't operate wort a sheet. I'm a not gonna let heem even cut da skeen ona one of my peoples, 'cause for chure he'll fook it up."

Howell, our mild-mannered spine guru, wasn't quite so harsh. "Well, he's not quite that bad Tano, but he certainly doesn't take instruction all that well. I've had to tell him several times not to use the bipolar cautery next to the nerve root, and he really is almost a menace with the drill anywhere around the spinal canal."

I'd come in at zero-dark-thirty several days earlier to watch Tim and Riley remove a large sub-dural hematoma in an elderly patient. The younger resident had done almost all of the case with Tim's assistance, and contrary to Tano's and Howard's comments, things had gone smoothly from skin to skin. No raised voices, curse words or slapped hands; the only slightly unusual thing was that Tim had stayed scrubbed right by Riley's side until the last stitch had been placed. I never even opened my mouth, other than to say hello, during the procedure. It was a nice, neat professional job, and I'd told them both so at the time, so now I asked Tim to weigh in on the debate.

"Well, Riley's not dumb and he doesn't have any physical problem that I can see, but he has a real hard time taking instructions- about anything. I checked, and English is his native language, but it's like he doesn't understand. Then, when you finally get pissed off because he's not doing whatever you've told him for the third time, his brain just turns into mush and nothing works. It's almost as if he doesn't have any mental structure to hang new information on, unless it's sorta chewed up for him in advance. I'm convinced he's trying-he's not a smart ass- he just doesn't know how."

The next morning in my office I re-played the discussion for Tim, then said, "This is one of the reasons I really want you to stay on with us. You're a fine teacher already and that's because, unlike most of us, it's not just your way or the highway. You're inside their heads- you resonate with how to get information across to these kids, even knuckleheads like Riley, and you've got the patience of a saint. This is a gift, buddy. Who are you going to use it on in private practice?"

Tim shook his head." I can't do it, boss. Standing there, watching somebody fumble with it- even in a nothing case like the other night- it eats me up. Even when they finally get it right -I'm happy for Riley, but my gut feels like it's been run through a wood chipper. God forbid he should ever hurt somebody while I'm helping him- I think I'd just shoot myself. I don't know how you do it, but forty years of that - even four years- would drive me around the bend. I'm going to have a hard-enough time living with my own screw-ups. Sincerely, I'm honored- but I'm going to pass."

So, it's not for everybody, but somebody has to do it. The ethical conflicts implicit in teaching one set of human beings to operate on another set of human beings should be obvious to even the most casual observer. In practice, they pose real dilemmas to surgeons, patients, students and to our larger society. At the heart of these conflicts is the apparent dichotomy between high quality patient care and excellent medical education, a dichotomy most marked in the clinical practice of a technically demanding, high risk surgical specialty like neurosurgery.

The fact that these very real conflicts have at least to date largely escaped rigorous examination by ethicists and philosophers is eloquent testimony to the efficacy of medicine's unobtrusive camouflage of its traditional teaching processes. More specifically, this paucity of scrutiny demonstrates how impenetrable a barrier the mystique of surgery has proven to be to lay examination. Without passing judgment at this point on the propriety of the deceit itself, I can say that in the current era in which there seems to be a presumed global right to all information, it will be surprising if this way of doing business persists.

The fragility of this veil of secrecy is highlighted by many of the writings of Atul Gawande, a surgeon and medical ethicist who first pointed out in 2002 the paradox between the imperative to provide patients the best possible care and the need to provide novice surgeons the experience necessary to become competent, independent operators. Gawande highlights the unpleasant fact that the skills, judgment and the confidence of which the mature surgeon is appropriately proud are all the results of hard- earned experience. Like the oboist, the team roper and the guy who repairs hard drives, we all have to practice to become good at what we do. There is one difference; in surgery, we practice on people.

As physicians, we generally find discussing this paradox with patients difficult, and understandably, patients definitely don't want to initiate the conversation. Yet, occasionally, potential patients will reveal their underlying anxieties by saying something like, "I don't want no intern operating on my brain." It's pretty hard to argue with that sentiment; given the stakes in neurosurgery, who in their right mind would agree to be "practiced on?"

A recent surgical patient myself, I can testify that while we're all in favor of both expertise and progress, when forced to a personal choice, we'll take expertise every time. If you don't believe that's correct, ask the residents what happens when an attending physician brings a family member into the hospital for an elective procedure. As the saying goes," This ain't no teaching case."

But teaching has to happen. The world at large refuses to acknowledge that operative excellence and educational progress are often mutually exclusive goals. Our society wants perfection without practice, but obviously everyone is harmed if we don't train the future generations of surgeons, which can't happen without a heightened patient exposure to errors, mistakes and false starts. Flying in the face of reality, one British report on public health stated:" There should be no learning curve as far as patient safety is concerned." What dream world is that?

This is the uncomfortable truth about surgery; you learn to operate by operating. Arrayed against that fact is unanimity in the public sphere that a patient's right to the best possible care must trump the training of the next generation of surgeons. In consequence there is an essential blanket of camouflage that covers much of surgical education, masking a system where operative experience must be appropriated, usually without consent, as a kind of bodily eminent domain.

The neurosurgeon/teacher walks a slippery slope as he or she struggles to honor personal and ethical commitments to patients, students, the society and to medicine itself . The resultant moral gymnastics are customized by each of us, but at one time or another we, each and all, are left feeling uneasy, unsatisfied, remorseful and perhaps even guilty by our individual solutions to the dilemmas imposed on us by real-life surgical instruction.

The surgeon's relationship with his or her patient, is a complex contract or covenant that leaves the physician responsible to the patient for what is generally described as 'reasonable and prudent care'. The physician is obligated to act toward the patient in such a fashion as to recognize her (the patient's) autonomy, promote her welfare, avoid injuring her and ensure that she receives the full benefits due her, as relates to her health, as a member of this society.

The explicit responsibilities a surgeon/ teacher accepts as regards his /her students are much less clearly defined, to the extent that any formal, consistent explanations are absent from both the medical and ethical literature. This is not a contractual relationship but rather a part of the code of conduct implicit in becoming a physician. As such it's not a reciprocal relationship, nor is it in any fashion legally binding on the teacher. Generally stated, the neurosurgeon has an obligation to encourage and promote the education of student neurosurgeons, and more subtly to share with them the information essential to preserving the highest possible quality of neurosurgical care for the community.

There is the additional unwritten implication that part of this duty is to identify and weed out those students either unfit or unqualified to practice medicine in general or this specialty in specific. Unfortunately, as our society becomes more politically correct, there is diminishing discussion about this unseemly but critical aspect of our responsibility to future patients.

Surprisingly, the ethical relationship between neurosurgeons and the society at large is detailed much more extensively than the student/ teacher relationship. In return for being permitted to practice medicine, the licensed neurosurgeon is admonished not to injure or abuse patients, to encourage a single high standard of medical practice, to abide by the laws of the country, to function as a physician advocate and to be involved in social activities especially as regards public health.

Finally, the neurosurgeon finds him or herself held subject to particular moral standards and restrictions by virtue of his/ her professional identity. In our own formal American code of ethics, the nature and scope of neurosurgical practice is defined, inappropriate personal conduct outlined and proscribed, dedication to furthering the fund of knowledge of the specialty is demanded and specific relationships with impaired physicians (and attorneys) outlined.

As variable as these relationships are, the conflict they infuse into our attempts to transform a young man or woman with five thumbs, two non-dominant hands, and a chronic inability to distinguish right from left into a competent neurosurgeon are very real. Before discussing my own approach to teaching, I thought it might be interesting to inspect the primary systems that have evolved in surgical education in terms of these conflicting demands. Oddball and eccentric systems aside, I think almost all neurosurgical training, at least in the US, can be assigned to one or a mixture of the following schemes.

Classical neurosurgical training in North America was patterned on the educational model developed in Great Britain and framed around the clinical practices of the surgical "greats", individuals like Harvey Cushing, Wilder Penfield, Walter Dandy and Henry Adson at institutions like the Mass General, Johns Hopkins, the Montreal Neurological Institute and the Mayo Clinic. In this system, as a rule the "boss" did all the big cases while 2-3 sub-bosses did the lesser stuff. "House officers", the student surgeons who would later come to be called residents, took care of patients on the wards, did most of the laboratory work, and assisted the big wheels during their operations.

Generally these residents worked in what came to be known as a pyramidal system, with a relatively large number (say 4-6) at the bottom and one survivor at the pinnacle after several years training and attrition. The last man standing was the "chief resident", the boss's designated boy, who scrubbed with the Great Man on all his cases, fetched his mail, and often picked him up in the morning and drove him home at night. This was the prized year of learning; not only did the "chief resident" get to be at the Chief's elbow at all times, but he also got to personally operate on any so-called "unfunded" or "charity" patients admitted to hospital with neurosurgery-type problems.

So, the substrate for basic technical surgical learning in most major institutions was the indigent patient population, a pattern we'll see again and again in surgical education. In this model, a given neurosurgery resident passively watched a lot of surgery and, even at the top of the pyramid, actually "did" a relatively modest amount. The real nuts and bolts of surgical technique were learned after leaving the nest, when the newly-minted surgeon ventured out on his own to practice on the unsuspecting public. A typical product of classical surgical training programs had seen "the master" do lots of cases but commonly had limited personal surgical experience. This classical teaching model has been referred to as the "Yes sir- No sir-Three bags full, sir" approach.

The other common training model, usually called "See one-Do one-Teach one ", developed almost exclusively in large city-county hospitals where again, almost exclusively, the patients were medically indigent; here they were said to "belong" to the resident staff. The amount of actual adult surgical activity – meaning that performed by certified, fully-trained neurosurgeons -varied between institutions. Of necessity there were some full-fledged neurosurgeons on each teaching hospital staff, but how much or how little they actually operated and / or supervised their residents was extraordinarily variable.

As a rule in these programs, the first year residents – the year following internship-were taught the basics of surgery by the second and third year guys, who in turn were instructed by the "senior" residents, all overseen by the chief resident, who personally operated on whatever he decided was a good case, often with minimal oversight. Consequently, these training programs tended to turn out surgeons with a surprising amount of individual operative experience, and more than abundant self- confidence but unfortunately, limited appreciation of many of the important variations, modifications and nuances of surgical practice and technique.

As a surgeon and a teacher, I think there are at least three different ways to decide where one fits into these two schemes. If you believe that every patient has the right to receive direct care from the most skilled, experienced surgeon in the building, and that the art of surgery can be learned at least as adequately by observing a good surgeon at work as by doing the work with one's own hands, then chances are you're going to be of the "Yes Sir-No Sir- Three Bags Full, Sir' school of education. On the other hand, if it's your opinion that surgical skills are relatively simple to acquire and, once acquired, can be polished by simple repetition on patients who don't know any better, you're probably a practicing advocate of the" See One-Do One- Teach One" method. Both of these models have been the main stream in American surgical education for the last 150 years.

A third approach, loosely based on five separate principles, has become relatively popular over the past three decades. This system modifies tenants of the two older methods and adds an original new concept. Those principles are as follows:

1. Every patient deserves care from a surgeon demonstrably competent to deal with his / her problem.
2. That care may or may not include the actual physical performance of her surgery.
3. A surgeon must physically perform an operation to master it.

4. Repetition is an essential element in surgical learning.
5. True understanding of any surgical procedure only comes with the ability to teach it.

This alternative concept involves recognition of the value of teaching to both the teacher and the student participating in the learning experience. In this hybrid system, an experienced surgeon assists an inexperienced surgeon who has previously demonstrated adequate technical skills in the performance of a "new" operation – one that is new to the assistant. The new guy, based on his operative performance, may perform all of the technical aspects of the case, only some of the procedure, or just a minimal amount; the teacher- who in fact may never touch the instruments- must be intellectually engaged for all of the portions of the procedure unfamiliar to the new guy. The value of this type instruction to the new guy is obvious. For the instructor, it's undeniable that the true test of understanding a surgical procedure is the ability to teach it to an appropriate student.

An outstanding neurosurgery resident, speaking to her mentor at the end of her seven-year training program, summed up the process like this:"So, first in the OR it was your hands and your head: then gradually it was my hands and your head; then it was my hands and my own head (with you in the background), and finally, it was someone else's hands and my head." That's the best summary of a successful neurosurgery training program ever written.

Despite sociological changes which pose conflicting demands on surgical training, the essence of learning to be an operator involves just doing the procedure; clumsy floundering around, moments of insight, the dawn of knowledge and ultimately the acquisition first of skill and then of confidence. Day after day, doing harder and harder tasks, each with increasing risks. Surgeons still learn by practicing on people; the rich, the poor, the uninsured, the VIP's mother, all alike. Students, teachers...and patients.

CHAPTER NINETEEN

The Good Surgeon

John Shepherd was an orthopedic spine surgeon, a Texas boy (by definition not a genius) with a big heart and a bigger smile, who doggedly slugged it out through medical school, residency and spine fellowship training. He ended up becoming a rising star in national orthopedics and was hired as the "spine expert" for the Orthopedics Department at our Medical Center. Both neurosurgeons and orthopedic surgeons do spine work, so most places there's a healthy tension between the two specialties. Before John arrived on the scene, the tension was unhealthy at our place because there was abundant evidence none of the Ortho guys were safe around the spinal canal, and I was happy to share that conclusion with anyone who showed an interest. So, when John was recruited I figured he was just another health hazard that needed to be avoided. I told him so one afternoon when he appeared uninvited in my office, asking for ten minutes of my time.

It was an important ask and the time (almost an hour) well spent for both of us. John started by telling me he had the utmost respect for neurosurgeons and had come by it the hard way. His father had suffered a near-fatal hemorrhage from an intra-cranial aneurysm, and throughout his illness,the surgeons' intensity and empathy had left a permanent positive impression on the young med student. Without blowing his own horn, John told me that was the same way he thought about patients. While he felt he might have something to contribute to our spine efforts, he knew for certain that he could learn a lot from our neurosurgeons, and he'd do anything to convince us of that fact.

John Shepherd was as good as his word, and over the next several years all of us (surgeons and patients alike) were graced by his contributions. There was nothing he wouldn't do to make patient care better; if that meant asking a neurosurgeon to operate on one of his own patients because the neuro guy had more experience or better luck with this type case or because John had blisters on his hands from operating on trauma all night, it didn't matter. He just wanted two things; the best for the patient, and an opportunity to learn for himself.

There wasn't much John couldn't do, but he definitely wasn't the slickest technical surgeon. I remember looking in on him doing a cervical laminectomy one afternoon, and over his shoulder telling him (and the whole OR) I thought he had the manual dexterity of a seal. He took it with a smile, then said something like," Yeah, but I usually do get the bleeding stopped." A none-too-subtle reference to the patient I was in the process of returning to the OR for a post-op clot.

John's surgical judgement was exquisite, never doing more than what the patient needed, always taking his time to get things "exactly right" but capable of being sudden and aggressive when the situation called for it. Post-op, long after the rest of us had headed for lunch or the office, he'd be in the OR Waiting Room, sitting down to talk with his patients' families, and he ended every day, no matter how late, with a swing through the ICU and ward to see his post-ops, even if they were really my patients and he's just lent a hand during their operations.

John Shepherd was the ultimate team player- the patient's team. When my frail, eighty-year-old mother needed a spinal decompression, I asked him and one of my partners to do it together; I have no idea who did what intra-operatively, but she made a spectacular recovery, and loved them both. John himself, and later in company with his young partner, made rounds with our spine guys, developed a joint weekly conference and switched residents back and forth like they were all family. It was the best of all situations, and far too good to last.

John Shepherd was a secret we couldn't keep; after a while a respected medical center in the Rocky Mountain West came calling with an offer we couldn't match. I wrote John the most elaborate letter of recommendation ever and when the neurosurgery chair there called to make sure I hadn't lost my mind, I convinced him to offer Dr. Shepard a joint appointment, knowing he would be a great asset to both departments . All of us shed a few tears at John's going-away celebration. Walking back to the office with my colleagues, I remember one of them saying, "Now, there's a really good surgeon- I don't care if he *is* a damn orthopedist."

Two years later on a Sunday morning, Patricia and I were out for a short jog when my infernal beeper went off. We hustled back home where the answering service had an urgent call from John's new medical institution. Greg Thomas, a stellar young vascular neurosurgeon, was calling to tell me John was in critical condition with a ruptured aneurysm. He also wanted me to know that John had told his wife that should that ever happen- as it had happened with his dad- he'd want me to operate on him. Greg Thomas was already one of the most outstanding cerebro-vascular surgeons in America; it was his hospital, his OR …and John Shepherd was already his friend. Greg wanted me to come, so I went.

There are lots of hurdles between a leisurely morning jog in Dallas and an emergency mid-afternoon craniotomy 1800 miles away, but we made it over most of them and through the rest. By the time I was scrubbed, Greg had John's head open ; in another thirty minutes or so, together we'd secured the aneurysm and cleaned out as much old blood as was safe. But what we saw wasn't hopeful. The aneurysm had ruptured straight up through the undersurface of the forebrain into the ventricular system, leaving the ventricles choked with clot. The clot was almost certain to produce hydrocephalus, but that could be treated; the big issue was the amount of damage to the mesial frontal lobes, where much of memory, a lot of problem solving and most rational thought lives. John would live, still be a good husband and a great father, but his life as a superb surgeon was over.

Over almost forty years, I've been blessed with the opportunity to know a large number of surgeons and the good fortune to have a hand in teaching over 100 young men and women how to do this work. It would be surprising if those experiences hadn't led me to think a lot about the make-up of a "good surgeon," a surgeon like John S. That designation is a little harder to earn from one's peers than you might think, in part because being a good surgeon is hard to define. Perhaps, as has been said about pornography, good surgeons are difficult to describe but easy to recognize, although I believe it's often easier to specify what they're not, as opposed to what they actually are. Let's try that route for starters. You can't be a bad doctor and a good surgeon. That's not just because the rules say you must first become a doctor before being a surgeon, but because surgery calls for the same intelligence, deep concern and empathy for patients that have been characteristics of the best physicians since there first were physicians. Compassion for the afflicted and a willingness to sacrifice oneself to relieve that misery are the infallible hallmarks of the true physician, whether she heals with medicine, laser beams, radiation or an amputation saw. There are some generic exceptions; for example, I don't know where "pure esthetic surgeons" fit into this categorization (although I'm pretty sure it's near the very bottom) but they damn sure have to be distinguished from real plastic surgeons like Paul Tessier and Jim Thornton. As I hope you'll see, it's not the hands but the heart and head that make the difference.

Dr. Ben Carson has gained a lot of attention with his autobiography, modestly entitled "Gifted Hands." I have no idea if Dr. Carson could actually operate his way out of a wet paper bag, but so-called "gifted hands" have very little to do with being a good surgeon, and probably not much to do with being a good surgical technician, which is a much different animal. To develop good surgical technique- cutting, sewing, manipulating, dissecting – basic manual dexterity is important, but surgical technique is a learned, and learnable, skill. In the absence of severe physical or neurological impairment- meaning if your eyes work together and you can assemble a cross word puzzle on your own - it's a skill that can be taught, practiced and continually improved. True technical virtuosity- the province of an extreme few (I've known two)-is the product of natural physical talents magnified by years of study and experience. It's wonderful to watch in real life or on tape, but its rarity simply magnifies the importance of the four qualities that truly make up the exceptional surgeon: thoughtfulness, judgment, situational awareness and personal honesty.

Bryce Michael has focused his career on patients with brain tumors for the past thirty-five years ; he enjoys operating on almost all of them, from the tiny hormone secreting tumors of the pituitary glad to the massive menigiomas of the skull base and the rare, shy lesions that grow silently submerged in CSF within the brain's ventricles. He's not such a big fan of the more common gliomas that arise from the stromal support cells of the brain itself, the so-called "low grade" gliomas that are only " sorta" malignant until they transform themselves into bad actors. His least favorites are the truly malignant glioblastomas which despite being hammered with everything in our arsenal still remain beyond cure. Bryce understands the habits and peculiarities of each of these tumors, the variable ways they present, spread, grow, and conceal themselves much like a seasoned fisherman distinguishes between the behavior of black bass and cutthroat trout. Looking at a time sequence of MRI studies, he can foresee a tumor's growth pattern, predict with startling accuracy where the next finger of bad news will show up and describe, almost down to the cellular level, what that brain- tumor interface will be like for the surgeon who must dissect the two apart. If you ask, he'll modestly even tell you the best surgical tool to use in that dissection.

This deep reservoir of clinical acumen underlies much of his analytical prowess. The rest stems from his personal knowledge of his patients and himself. Unlike many of us, Bryce has made the conscious decision to immerse himself in his patients' lives, to come to know their families, hopes, aspirations, and especially their fears. Many surgeons will never realize that, for some patients, what *can* be done- in the objective management of their disease- isn't necessarily what *should* be done for the whole patient. Tumor surgeons especially confront a tremendous amount of misfortune destined to engulf many patients and their families; finding the "right' role for a surgeon to play in each case is a difficult task, one that's impossible if the players don't trust you sufficiently to open their hearts.

During my own career I frequently did this aspect of the job poorly, in part as a selfish protection against being hurt, but primarily to prevent emotional paralysis the next time I had to face a similar situation. Bryce has quietly taken the other track, softly but strongly embracing his patents -not just their diseases but their humanity -for the long haul. As a result, he and his wife Barbara, who's also a surgeon, have been honored guests at more patient weddings, christenings and yes, funerals, than the entire rest of our institution's large faculty. Bryce goes to the OR knowing, not just the tumor, but the human cursed with carrying it.

The other important component of Bryce's judgment rests in his self-awareness. By this point in his career, he's operated in the ballpark of 5,000 brain tumors; while he doesn't claim to recall every one, he's not shy about the composite lessons he has learned from the experience. Some of that is the stuff you'd expect, characteristics of the tumors, like consistency, vascularity, rigidity, etc. However, the deciding portion of those lessons relate to his own capabilities; the pluses and minuses in his operative abilities that have influenced the outcomes of operations on this specific tumor, on tumors of this size, in or near this location, with this type margin, in patients of this age and this health, in patients with this set of post-op needs and expectations. And amazingly, Bryce can and will share those thoughts with you – on the spot- if you ask. It's one of his greatest talents both as a surgeon and a teacher. This open self- awareness precludes secrets, vanity and ego. Which is by no means the routine description of a brain surgeon.

As neurosurgeons, most of us can and do brag (almost ceaselessly) about our wizardry in getting ourselves (and our patients) out of really tough spots. Without question, being able to answer the bell when the feces get in the fan is an important surgical skill. However, the best complications are those you avoid, and keeping the plumbing metaphors at bay requires a continuous awareness of "where am I", and "what comes next". Knowing in real time how the tumor/ mass/ aneurysm has distorted the normal anatomy, how the tissues "feel", what tension the objects being dissected are under, and always- what's the emergency protocol if, all of a sudden, things go south.

This type of situational awareness is a difficult skill to master and frequently a harder one to maintain. Neurosurgical operations tend to be very long, during which time the surgeon's focus is continually on a highly magnified, brilliantly lit area, while everything on the periphery is small, out of focus or completely hidden. In addition, the problems inherent in just doing the job at hand tend to crowd out other considerations, things like what's hiding behind that sliver of bone or what will happen if I just put a little more traction on this brain retractor or can I tug on this nerve/vessel/ tumor a skosh harder? Throughout any protracted case, there are multiple distractions- emotional, intellectual and physical- but if the surgeon can't keep his head out of his butt and on a swivel until the show's over, he becomes an increasing liability to his patient as the day grows longer.

Bryce shares many of his long cases with another surgeon, most commonly an ENT specialist, who will do the opening for pituitary lesions or large tumors at the skull base. It's instructive to watch Bryce when he takes over to do the actual tumor removal. First, regardless of what's gone before, he'll check the functionality of his instruments; what's the vacuum setting on both suctions? Does the bipolar cautery work and how hot is it? Is the brain retractor ready and its tension bar set correctly? Are the cottonoids nice and wet and does the scrub have some Gelfoam strips in the sizes he likes?

Then, he'll simply sit at the microscope inspecting the operative field for several minutes without an instrument in his hand. He's memorizing the unique anatomy, comparing what he sees (and what he doesn't see) with the preliminary operative map in his head, updating the template he'll use as a backdrop to the tumor resection. Next, using the instruments very gently, he'll tell himself about the tactile status of the operative field, learning how the vessels feel, the amount of slack in each nerve, whether the brain is soft or tense or wet or dry, the tumor's consistency, the vessels on its surface, its degree of adherence to the normal brain and /or the dura, and its potential dissection planes. He's in no hurry to begin. Here, slow is smooth and smooth is safe.

The final critical characteristic of the good surgeon is personal honesty. There are multiple aspects of that trait important to the would-be patient. Does your surgeon take the time and make the effort to teach you about your problem, about its anatomy and the issues involved in its surgical resolution? Does she tell you straight-forwardly about her own experience, or does she quote you success rates and complications from the latest publication written by some Swiss master who's 85 years old and has done half a million? Does he explain exactly who's going to do what in the OR? Will he be there all the time, some of the time or just "available by telephone" to the guys doing the work-and who *are* those guys? Depending on the nature of your problem, there are several reasonable answers to these questions, all of which are better known prior to the operation than learned later. Finally, do you believe she (your potential surgeon) really knows your name, or are you just another box she's checking on the way to riches and /or stardom?

Bryce approaches these issues something like this in his pre-op discussions:

"I've done about X of these in my career, and most but certainly not all of my patients have done well. The last time we totaled these numbers a couple of years back, about Y % of patients were able to return to full activity within six months. The risk of you dying because of the operation is about Z% and another M% of patients will suffer some long-term disability. We've already talked in the clinic about those specific potential complications; I don't believe you'll fall in this category, but there is always that risk.

"You've already met Lisa here, our outstanding resident. She'll scrub with me on your case and will do some of the operation, with me standing right there for guidance. The more difficult or risky parts of the procedure will be all mine, and I won't leave the operating room until every bit of the surgery except the simple closure are finished. At that time, I'll come out to the waiting room to tell your folks how things have gone, and then I'll be in my office next door watching Lisa on TV as she finishes up.

What I can promise you is that I'll do my very best-all of us will. I believe you've made the right choice to have this operation and I also believe this is going to work out well."

That's what a patient should hear- and believe.

I realize that a patient searching for a doctor, a department chairman looking for a new surgeon, or a hospital administrator shopping for a new "revenue stream" all will have great difficulty judging potential applicants on the basis of these criteria. Knowledge, judgement, situational awareness and personal honesty are tough to evaluate on a website or in an advertisement but talking with other patients, doctors and nurses can provide some important insight. Learning if "the guy" has a regional or national reputation can be of help, and the National

Physicians' Data Base can serve as an early warning alert to past problematic issues. There's no one sure way, but on the other hand, the process as outlined probably isn't any harder than trying to determine if your would-be surgeon has "gifted hands".

CHAPTER TWENTY

Rules

The Good Surgeon's Rules of Engagement

- Recognize that all surgical risks involve someone else's life.
- Understand that some of your most successful operations will be those you choose not to do.
- Be more familiar with your surgical limitations than with your bank account.
- Realize the most you can promise a patient is that you'll do your best.
- Never quote another surgeon's "numbers" (risks, complications, success rates) as your own.
- Always ask yourself, "If this, then what?" Or- "What's my plan when the shit hits the fan?"
- Someone else should do any potential operation you haven't thought through at least twice
- Never trust the diagnosis sent with a transfer or referral. If the guys on the other end were so smart they wouldn't need to transfer the patient
- Always interpret your own images. X-rays are uniformly correct; radiologists not so much.

- Remember: re-operations are twice as difficult, twice as bloody, twice as complicated and twice as risky.
- Never be late to the OR. It's the sure sign of a self- centered horse's ass.
- On your way to the OR, don't pass the Surgeon's Restroom without making a contribution.
- Good anesthesiologists are God's gift to fallible surgeons. Treat them with the utmost respect.
- Always position your own operative patients
- Always have one more suction available than you think you'll need.
- Never turn on any device in the OR that you must turn off to deal with the inevitable emergency.
- Idle chatter in the OR is a diversion most patients can't afford
- Don't guess about anatomy; always show it to yourself.
- Proximal control is the golden rule. Distal control is icing on the cake.
- If your scrub nurse is reluctant to pass you a particular instrument, it's probably not what you need.
- Surgical temper tantrums are like dirty diapers; all that shit demonstrates is a dismal lack of self-control.
- If it helps to say, "fuck" occasionally, say it. Then apologize.
- Calculate your estimated blood loss, double it, and then add 10%. That'll get you in the ballpark.
- Never leave the OR without saying "Thank You "to the scrub and circulating nurses.
- Change your scrubs before talking to the family; you're their doctor, not their butcher.
- When an ICU nurse tells you a patient "just isn't right", you've got an upcoming disaster.
- Good surgeons are slow to take patients to the OR but quick to take them back.
- Don't stay too long at the dance.